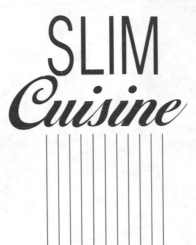

SLIM
Cuisine

Sue Kreitzman
and the Editors of Consumer Reports Books

CONSUMER REPORTS BOOKS
A DIVISION OF CONSUMERS UNION
Yonkers, New York

LIBRARY OF CONGRESS CATALOGING-IN-PUBLICATION DATA

Kreitzman, Sue.
Slim cuisine : innovative techniques for healthful cooking / Sue
Kreitzman and the editors of Consumer Reports Books.
p.   cm.
Includes index.
ISBN 0-89043-187-6
1. Reducing diets—Recipes.   2. Low-fat diet—Recipes.   3. Low-
calorie diet—Recipes.   I. Consumer reports.   II. Title.
RM222.2.K7   1991
641.5′63—dc20   90-24458
CIP

Design by Kathryn Parise

First printing, May 1991
Manufactured in the United States of America

Slim Cuisine is a Consumer Reports Book published by Consumers Union, the non-profit organization that publishes *Consumer Reports*, the monthly magazine of test reports, product Ratings, and buying guidance. Established in 1936, Consumers Union is chartered under the Not-for-Profit Corporation Law of the State of New York.

The purposes of Consumers Union, as stated in its charter, are to provide consumers with information and counsel on consumer goods and services, to give information on all matters relating to the expenditure of the family income, and to initiate and to cooperate with individual and group efforts seeking to create and maintain decent living standards.

To ANH

CONTENTS

ACKNOWLEDGMENTS

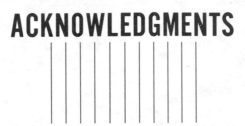

As an American living and working in England, I am extremely grateful to my new friends in England, particularly the readers of my Slim Cuisine books and the viewers of my BBC television spots who have helped to make the last six years of my life such happy and productive ones.

Without my staff—Rosemarie Espley, Sandie Perry, Brenda Huebler, and Mary Hardy—I would not accomplish a fraction of what I do. They are like a second family to me, and make my working life a great pleasure.

Alan Howard and The Howard Foundation have had faith in my particular philosophy of weight maintenance since 1982. They make it possible for me to continue developing Slim Cuisine to its full potential.

My "foodie spies" back home, especially Margaret and Terry Pedersen, keep me up-to-date—between trips home—on low-fat food product development in the United States.

Gail Piazza, a consultant for *Consumer Reports*, has worked hard testing and retesting the Slim Cuisine recipes and techniques.

And my family, as always, provides emotional support, love, and unlimited *fun!*

Thanks to all of you!

1

Slim Cuisine
Basics

INTRODUCTION

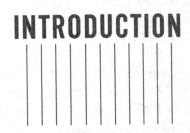

My Fattening Career

As a cook, my mother was worse than mediocre. From its taste and texture, her beef stew seemed to be prepared with bargain cuts of dinosaur, and the less said about the greasy gravy, the better. I grew up with little inkling of the sensuality and comforting nature of food and, as a result, was a relatively slim child and teenager. I didn't know that some people ate for the pleasure of it, and not merely because their mothers insisted on it. But then I grew up. I attained my own kitchen (it soon became my favorite room). I began, slowly, to learn the truths of the gastronomic universe. It was the early 1960s, and the little ethnic restaurants of New York were my classrooms; their proprietors were my first cooking teachers, along with the butchers and greengrocers in my own neighborhood of Washington Heights, who were always patient with my endless questions.

By the early 1970s, I knew that I had a talent, undetected in my early years, for food appreciation and for cooking. By 1972, I had become a full-fledged food professional, and it was abundantly evident that I had an additional (related) talent—for gaining weight. From 1962—when it all began in my small but beloved New York kitchen—to 1982—when I operated a cooking school, a restaurant review newsletter, and a thriving food-writing career from my large Atlanta, Georgia, kitchen—I spiraled from 130 pounds to 215 pounds. It wasn't a steady climb. The escalation began in 1962, when I discovered the seductive nature of food. The next twenty years were a series of ups and downs (mainly ups) while I struggled: Life was a constant attempt to balance pleasure (eating) and denial (dieting), and pleasure usually won, although guilt—when my weight would drop slightly, only to rebound higher than ever—was a constant companion.

In 1982, circumstances came to the rescue. As the director of the Center for Nutritional Health at a large university, my husband, Dr. Stephen Kreitzman (a Ph.D. in nutritional biochemistry), was about to conduct a study testing the safety and efficacy of a VLCD (very low Calorie diet). Distressed at my ever-increasing weight and my endlessly burgeoning figure, I volunteered to be one of his study subjects. On a VLCD, one consumes a nutrition-rich, Calorie-shy formula three times a day. *That's all*, except for enough water to float a small tanker. Several months later I emerged from this stringent regime a reborn slim person; there, at last, was the willowy waist of my teen years, the cheekbones, the firm chin line, all the lovely slim parts I thought I'd never see again. But my joy was clouded by harsh facts; were I to hurl myself back into my well-established buttery, creamy, oily habits, I would soon be saying hello again to a billowing backside, bulging tummy, double chin, and quivering thighs.

I was determined to indulge *both* my passions: my love of food *and* my burning desire to remain slim. Slim Cuisine is the direct result: a maintenance cuisine that enables the cook to produce tantalizing and delicious dishes that are low in Calories (especially empty Calories and fat Calories), high in nutrition, yet very delicious and comforting. Slim Cuisine is based on new techniques of cooking that do not depend on fats or oil, as the old techniques do. Imagine: ice cream, fried potatoes, Italian sausages, lasagna, hamburgers—yet the willowy waist does not expand and the cheekbones remain visible. Oh, Brave New World!

The basic premise of Slim Cuisine is that dietary fat must go. At more than twice the number of Calories per gram as carbohydrates and proteins, fat is a significant contributor to obesity. Even worse, it is considered to be one of the major cardiac risks. And, in addition to heart and blood vessel disease, it has been linked to several kinds of cancer. Saturated animal fat is not the only culprit. There are health problems with monounsaturated and polyunsaturated fats, too. And it doesn't matter if you're cooking with butter, margarine, sunflower oil, yak fat, or blubber—it still has a dense 9 Calories per gram (well over 120 Calories per *tablespoon!*)—and these Calories go straight to your hips with deadly efficiency.

The American Heart Association recommends a dietary fat level of no more than 30 percent of total Calories. The pioneering cooking techniques used in Slim Cuisine bring the fat levels down to below that point, yet retain the ravishing richness that foodies crave.

The recipes are Calorie and fat shy, yet nutrient dense. Sugar and salt have been drastically reduced, too, yet there is enough taste and texture to knock your socks off. Some recipes are for family-type meals, others are for elegant entertaining. There is plenty of so-called junk food—hamburgers, fries, pizza, and ice cream—and there is plenty of delicious ethnic food—Italian, Indian, Mexican, Chinese . . . And the best news is this: If you have been living on a high-fat diet and switch to Slim Cuisine, you will *lose* weight painlessly and happily.

FAMILY FEEDING

Slim Cuisine is for the whole family. Don't make a big fuss explaining to other members of the household how low in fat and dietetic the recipes are. If they wonder why you are cooking these wonderful new recipes all of a sudden, simply explain that you are taking up a new hobby: gourmet cooking. These recipes taste *nothing* like that awful four-letter word (*diet*). What family members don't know, won't hurt them—indeed, it will help them.

Children, who should not diet and who should not be on extremely low-fat diets, can have extras: semiskimmed milk and semiskimmed products; dried fruit; low-sugar, nonfat baked beans—but I firmly believe that children *never* need junk food, such as potato chips, fried foods, candy, store-bought cakes, doughnuts, and so on.

ESSENTIAL FATTY ACIDS

A totally fat-free diet would be almost impossible to achieve. No one should even attempt such a diet; it would be dangerous. A certain amount of essential fatty acids are necessary each day to maintain health. There is no need to worry about fatty acid levels in the Slim Cuisine regime. The vegetables, grains, fish, meats, and poultry you will be consuming contain more than enough of these essential fats. *Added* fats are not necessary. This is not just a guess or wishful conjecture. All Slim Cuisine recipes have been computer-analyzed. Further checking was done by sending samples of many cooked recipes to an independent laboratory for analysis. The fatty acids necessary for good health were shown to be present in ample quantity.

Weight Maintenance

Foodies are fascinated, delighted, and comforted by food. They expect cuisine to be rich, compelling, and delicious and they want portions to be generous. Even FFFs (Formerly Fat Foodies) like me want food to conform to these standards. Although we long to stay slim, we still crave plenty of good things to eat. I mean *really* good things. A leaf of lettuce, a naked morsel of broiled fish, and a steamed vegetable do little to assuage our cravings. We want sauces, we want creamy textures, we want glamour, we even want, occasionally, junk food. What to do? Periods of abstinence followed by periods of indulgence are unhealthy and frustrating. Tiny portions of luscious things cause agony.

Calorie counting and continuous deprivation in the name of slimness is sheer hell, and difficult as well. Don't let this problem compromise your physical and mental health, or your sensual enjoyment of food. Be very careful. Don't fall into the three major weight-maintenance traps.

TRAP #1: FOOD OBSESSION

Food obsession occurs when one constantly worries about what one eats, counts every Calorie, and checks the scale several times a day for added pounds. Pleasure in food becomes forbidden, feared, and longed for at the same time. Occasionally lapses occur. Fraught with guilt, the diner gorges on unsuitable, unhealthy, and fattening foods, only to diet austerely for several days afterward to make up for the transgression. This behavior results in an extremely unhealthy and nutritionally unbalanced diet and an anxious mental state.

TRAP #2: THE MATH-MAJOR SYNDROME

If you are determined to eat nutritious food, to balance your diet properly, and to ingest every Calorie, every micro and macro nutrient in perfect harmony according to your needs, you may find yourself a slave to your calculator and to nutritional tables. Every meal becomes an intricate math exercise, as you work out protein levels, vitamins, minerals, and trace minerals. Mealtimes are grim accounting sessions, and soon they become so boring that you toss your calculator away and fling yourself into bad eating habits again.

TRAP #3: THE YO-YO SYNDROME

The initial joy and novelty of newly lost weight slowly wears off as food's siren song becomes louder and louder. It's so easy to fall back into the bad old habits. After all, if you eat that gooey chocolate cream cake, devour a jumbo order of greasy French fries, succumb to oceans of hollandaise, mountains of fudge, butter-slathered biscuits, why, you can always go back on your diet for a few days, can't you? Soon you find yourself eating mindlessly again, no thought at all for nutrition and Calories, until your clothes are embarrassingly tight and you can't stand the sight of your puffy face in the mirror anymore. Then the struggle starts again. The yo-yo syndrome can last a lifetime.

Slim Cuisine Forever

Slim Cuisine is the answer. Don't ever think about going "on" a diet, no matter how fiercely you long to get trim. Going "on" a diet implies that eventually you are going to go "off" again. And once you switch "off" you'll find what 95 percent of all dieters who have managed to shed pounds have found. *Losing* the weight was relatively easy, *keeping* it off is well-nigh impossible. And often, if you have gone "on" a diet, only eventually to go "off" again, it's not just a matter of regaining the lost weight; it may come back with even more poundage than you lost in the first place.

Use Slim Cuisine, my low-fat method of cooking, to keep slim and happy. You may use it for weight loss *and* lifetime weight maintenance, or you may use it as the next step, when you have lost a considerable amount of weight on a VLCD or any other diet regime. If you leap from such a regime into your old habits again, all your hard work will have been futile. If, on the other hand, you ease into Slim Cuisine, you will maintain your weight loss for a lifetime. Just remember, food is meant to be wonderful. When life turns sour, food is there to console us; when fortune smiles, food is there to help us celebrate. It nourishes, comforts, and provides sensuality and fun in equal measure. Slim Cuisine provides the comfort, the celebration, and the sensuality without the usual accompaniments of guilt and fat. It is a safe harbor for those who struggle with being overweight and have a guilt-ridden relationship with food. And the new habits you learn will last a lifetime.

A NOTE ON CALORIE AND FAT COUNTS

Calorie counting is boring and self-defeating. When you worry too much about such things, you ruin your eating pleasure, and you may find yourself cutting down too much out of fear of Calories. Because Slim Cuisine cuts out so much fat, the Calorie levels in my recipes are very low in general. Nevertheless, I couldn't resist including some here and there so you could join me in gloating over the astonishing difference between Slim Cuisine recipes and the traditional versions.

It is important to eat lavishly to keep your nutrients and morale high. Use Slim Cuisine techniques religiously, do not succumb to wicked outside temptations, use your common sense, and you will lose weight in a very well fed manner—without counting Calories.

YIELDS

One of the important points of Slim Cuisine is that large portions are permissible. And—in general—a portion is not a portion is not a portion. One person's portion is another person's tantalizing tease and yet another person's overindulgence. It is Slim Cuisine policy to allow you the delicious freedom to decide for yourself what constitutes a portion according to the occasion and the diners. That is why, whenever possible, the yield is given in volume (for instance, 3 cups) or in pieces (24 meatballs). Because the fat density is drastically diminished and Calorie counting is eliminated, portion control is no longer necessary.

TECHNIQUES

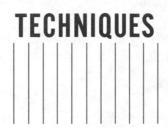

The new techniques described in this book will enable you to produce rich, satisfying, and comforting food without the excess Calories and fat. All Slim Cuisine recipes are nutrient dense, Calorie shy, and exceedingly palatable. Here is a brief overview of the basic rules.

1. Dispense with all cooking fats and oils. It doesn't matter if the fats are unsaturated (monounsaturated or polyunsaturated) or saturated; dump them all and forget about them for the rest of your life. The no-no list includes:

Butter
Margarine and "low-fat" spreads
Drippings, lard, schmaltz, suet, poultry fats
Poultry skin
All oils: sunflower, olive, peanut, corn, soybean, et cetera
Solid hydrogenated shortenings
Mayonnaise and salad dressings
All dairy products not made from skim milk with the exception of two medium-fat cheeses: Parmesan and part-skim mozzarella, which may be used in recipes occasionally in small quantities.

High-fat meats

Nuts, except for a very small amount here and there for flavoring and garnishing, and except for chestnuts, which are very low in fat.

Whole eggs only very occasionally. The yolk is quite high in fat. The whites, on the other hand, are fat-free; use them as often as you please.

Baked goods and prepared foods containing any of the above fats or high-fat ingredients.

2. Use the following as substitutes for the forbidden fats:

Skim milk yogurt. Use it as is or drain it to make a substitute for cream cheese or a base for Slim "Mayonnaise" and salad dressings (see pages 21–22).

Skim milk fromage blanc or fromage frais, if they are available in your area. Use as described for yogurt and also in place of sour cream and crème fraîche (see pages 21–22).

Buttermilk cultured from skim milk

Skim milk cottage cheese

Skim milk quark, if it is available in your area (see page 38).

Skim milk and skim milk powder

✓ Chicken, beef, and vegetable stocks (see pages 31–35). Use very good quality stock in place of butter and oil to sauté and flavor vegetables (see page 14).

Lean meats, poultry trimmed of skin and fat

3. Use vegetables that have been baked and then puréed to give body to sauces, casseroles, stews, soups, and gratins (see pages 23–29). The best vegetables for this purpose are garlic, onions, carrots, potatoes, parsnips, rutabagas, and turnips.

4. Use baked, puréed eggplant (see page 28) as a filler in meatballs, hamburgers, meat sauce, and so on. It gives body and moisture, cuts down on the amount of meat used, and adds no eggplant taste. Purée roasted and peeled peppers, season, and use as a nonfat, delicious sauce for pasta, meats, fish, or poultry.

5. Don't give up desserts, only those that are laden with fat and excessive sugar. For instance, ice cream, that high-fat, sugary disaster,

becomes low-fat, low-Calorie, and highly nutritious made the Slim Cuisine way (see page 222).

Some Slim Cuisine techniques—the ones you will use over and over again—are detailed in this section. Other more specific techniques—stir-frying without oil, for instance, or ridding meat of fat— are outlined in the appropriate chapters.

I hope that these techniques will enable you to think about cooking in an entirely new way. Make them part of your culinary life; substitute them for the old high-fat methods and you will be cutting hundreds, even thousands, of Calories out of your day's intake. One of the most exciting results of this kitchen revolution is that you will be able to increase the amount of food you ingest each day.

The comforting thing about Slim Cuisine is the flexibility it gives to your everyday cooking. You can use many of your old recipes; in fact you can try new ones from intriguing new cookbooks. Just apply these techniques in place of traditional ones and you will be safe from the fat demons that lurk in conventional cooking. If a recipe calls for onions sautéed in butter or oil for instance, substitute Slim Cuisine Sautéed Onions. Use baked garlic purée instead of minced garlic sautéed in oil, fromage blanc or yogurt cheese in place of sweet or sour cream, Slim Cuisine "Mayonnaise" in place of the very wicked real thing. You will save thousands of Calories, yet eating and exploring the world of cuisine will continue to be a joyous activity.

Remember, when following any recipe, make your kitchen life easier by first reading the recipe through completely and then having all the ingredients chopped, sliced, diced, poured, measured, et cetera, before you begin. Set the prepared ingredients out on your work surface along with any equipment needed. Only *then* should you begin the actual cooking.

Key to the Symbols

Slim Cuisine can be used for both weight loss *and* weight maintenance. And as with all cooking regimes, some recipes are fast, some complicated; some can be frozen, some call for a microwave; et cetera. To make your cooking life easier, the following symbols have been used when appropriate throughout the book:

☆ *Star* Everyone needs an occasional Therapeutic Binge—an opportunity to eat all they want of something delicious without fear of dire consequences (galloping fat, burgeoning flab, high blood pressure, clogged arteries). If a recipe is marked with a ☆, it is a Therapeutic Binge; eat *all you want* of that particular dish, anytime you want it.

♡ *Heart* These are very low fat recipes, and very low in sugar as well. If you wish to lose weight yet stay well-nourished, confine yourself to these recipes.

🕘 *Clock* A clock indicates a fast recipe, perfect for those days when you come home late, there is nothing prepared in the freezer, and you want something wonderful to eat. Some of the 🕘 recipes are elegant enough for guests. Some are homey, family-type recipes.

❄ *Snowflake* Snowflaked recipes are suitable for freezing.

▣ *Microwave* Many recipes call for a microwave oven. Some recipes are followed by microwave adaptations. Such recipes and footnotes are marked with ▣.

♙ *Chef's Toque* Recipes marked with a chef's toque take a bit more preparation than usual. These recipes are not *difficult*, merely somewhat more time-consuming. In all cases, the results are more than worth it.

Sautéing in Stock

Think about the way many recipes begin: "Sauté onions and/or garlic in 4 (or more) tablespoons oil or butter." Follow such directions and immediately, without even thinking, you add at least 480 fat Calories to the meal. Of course, it is usually much more than 480. Other recipes in the same meal may begin with similar directions. Add to this the recipes prepared for the other meals of the day—butter or margarine spread on bread, fried foods, high-fat snacks, melted butter on vegetables, mayonnaise on sandwiches, et cetera,—and the day's intake of fat Calories can easily mount to well over 1,000, without any effort at all. Begin your Slim Cuisine kitchen revolution by changing the sauté method from a fat-based one to a stock-based one.

It is important to realize that merely boiling or simmering onions in stock result in *flabby* vegetables, not *sautéed* vegetables. My technique combines onions and/or other vegetables with stock in a way that achieves a caramelized, deeply flavored *sautéed* effect.

SAUTÉED ONIONS

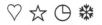 61 Calories per 1 large sautéed onion
0.2g fat
(Traditional sautéed onions:
250 Calories per 1 large
sautéed onion, 24g fat)

This is the basic technique. Chopped carrots and celery can be added. The best pot to use is an 8-inch enameled cast-iron frying pan. Do *not* use a nonstick frying pan. The intense flavor that results from this method depends upon a little judicious and controlled burning, occurring toward the end of the recipe. Don't even think about substituting a bouillon cube for homemade stock. The cube is loaded with salt, monosodium glutamate, and other undesirables and has no place in Slim Cuisine. (See pages 31–35 for recipes and hints about stock.)

1 large onion, chopped	Splash of dry vermouth, dry red
1 clove garlic, minced	or white wine, dry sherry, wine
¾ cup stock	vinegar, or additional stock

1. Combine first three ingredients in an 8-inch frying pan. Cover and bring to a boil.

2. Uncover and boil for approximately 5 minutes, until most of the

liquid has evaporated. Reduce heat and simmer until just about dry and beginning to stick a little bit.

3. Reduce heat again and toss, stirring constantly with a wooden spoon until you smell a lovely, toasty, oniony aroma and the bottom of the pan is beginning to brown just a bit. Pour in a splash of dry wine or additional stock and raise the heat again. Stir with the wooden spoon, scraping up all the browned bits. When the liquid is gone, the onions should be meltingly tender and amber-colored, and the tantalizing smell should be driving all members of the household mad. Remove from heat. Use in a recipe at once, or refrigerate or freeze for later use.

BROWNED ONIONS

           Makes about 2 cups

This makes the most delicious concoction imaginable. It is what the French call onion jam or onion marmalade. This Slim Cuisine version can save you many Calories, yet the final result is just as good as the sinful versions, if not more so.

6 large onions, peeled and trimmed 2 cups stock 3 to 4 tablespoons additional	stock, dry vermouth, dry red or white wine, dry sherry, or wine vinegar

1. Cut onions in half. Slice into thin half-moons. Combine onions and stock in a deep 10-inch enameled cast-iron frying pan. Cover and bring to a boil. Reduce heat a bit and simmer briskly for 10 minutes.

2. Uncover and simmer for 35 to 40 minutes, stirring occasionally. After this period of time the onions will be turning amber-brown and the liquid will be almost gone. Stir constantly and allow to cook for a few minutes more. The onions will begin to stick just a bit. Keep stirring for approximately 10 minutes more, until the onions are just about dry and browned bits are forming on the bottom of the frying pan. As you stir with your wooden spoon, keep scraping up the browned bits.

3. Raise the heat a tiny bit and let the onions start to burn just a *little*—that's what makes the ravishing flavor. Be very careful not to allow wholesale burning and blackening.

4. Splash in 3 to 4 tablespoons dry wine, wine vinegar, or additional stock. Boil until just about dry, vigorously stirring and scraping up the browned bits on the bottom of the frying pan. Immediately remove from heat. Use a rubber spatula to scrape the mass of browned onions into a storage container. Use as a garnish for lean meats, as a base for stews, sauces, and soups, or serve as a vegetable accompaniment.

ONION-HERB INFUSION

   Makes about ⅔ cup

This is another way of using onions and stock (scallions or shallots this time) to make an intensely flavored base for many recipes. Please note that in this method and the previous one the wine is boiled dry so no alcohol (and no alcohol Calories) are left. The herb you choose for the infusion will depend upon how you wish to use it. Tarragon, oregano, thyme all work beautifully with this method.

1½ cups sliced scallions (both green and white portions) or finely chopped shallots or onions
½ cup stock
½ cup dry vermouth or dry red or white wine

1 or 2 pinches cayenne pepper, or to taste
2½ tablespoons chopped fresh herbs, or 1½ teaspoons dried
1 tablespoon chopped fresh parsley

Combine all ingredients in a small heavy frying pan. Bring to a boil, reduce heat, and simmer briskly, uncovered (approximately 10 minutes), until almost all the liquid has evaporated. Use at once in a recipe or refrigerate or freeze for later use.

SAUTÉED ONIONS FOR CURRIES

♡ ☆ ⏰ ❄

Curries present a challenge. Indian cooking depends very heavily on ghee (clarified butter) or oil. The myriad spices and herbs that make up the flavoring mix for each curry must be gently cooked in the fat or oil. Sometimes herbs or spices are whole, sometimes ground, or sometimes pounded to a paste with garlic, ginger, and onions, but in whatever form they are always gently fried early in the recipe. It is this important step that gives Indian food its distinctive taste and texture. Just adding the appropriate spice mix to a fatless version of the recipe results in a finished dish with a sandy, gritty texture and a harsh, raw-spice taste: unpleasant to eat, and very un-Indian as well. Frying the spices dry in a nonstick pan scorches them. I've finally worked out a way to "fry" the spices with onions, ginger, and garlic in a way that produces a smooth, gentle effect, with no scorching, and in which all the seasonings blend well and leave no harshness. As is typical in Indian cooking, each curry recipe in this book has its own spice mix.

3 onions, chopped, sliced, or cut into eighths 1¼ cups stock	Chopped or minced garlic Spice mixture (see individual curry recipes for specifics)

1. Separate the segments of the chopped onion pieces and spread them in a heavy, nonstick frying pan. Add *no* liquid or fat. Heat the frying pan gently. Cook at moderate heat, without stirring, for 7 to 10 minutes, until the onions are sizzling, speckled with dark amber, and beginning to stick to the pan.

2. Stir in the stock and let it bubble up, stirring up the browned bits in the pan with a wooden spoon as it bubbles. Stir in the spices and garlic. Reduce the heat a bit and simmer, stirring frequently, until the mixture is very thick (not at all soupy), and the onions and spices are "frying" in their own juices. Don't rush this step; it is essential that the spices should not have a raw, harsh taste. Taste and cook very gently for a few more minutes, if necessary.

3. If you wish, for a thick sauce, purée half the mixture in a blender or food processor, then combine the puréed mixture with the unpuréed portion.

To this basic onion-curry mixture add more stock or chopped tomatoes or tomato paste. Stir in cubed meat, poultry, vegetables, shrimp or fish, and simmer until done. At the very end, yogurt may be added to the sauce.

Note: This basic method is correct for chili con carne, goulashes, and other dishes made with paprika, as well as curry.

SWEET-AND-SOUR ONIONS

Makes about 2 cups

These rich onions are perfect as a topping for meats—braised liver, grilled steak, hamburgers, et cetera—but they are very good on their own as well. (See page 97 for the lowest-fat steaks.)

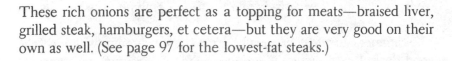

6 large onions, peeled	1 tablespoon sugar
½ cup stock	2 cloves garlic, crushed
½ teaspoon Dijon mustard	1 dried bay leaf, broken in half
1½ tablespoons red wine vinegar	Salt to taste

1. Slice onions into ½-inch-thick rings. Place in a nonreactive frying pan with the remaining ingredients.
2. Bring to a boil, reduce heat, cover, and simmer for 30 minutes, uncovering to stir occasionally.
3. Remove the cover and simmer, stirring until the onions are beautifully browned and the liquid has greatly reduced. Remove the bay leaf before serving.

SAUTÉED MUSHROOMS

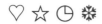

Makes about ½ cup

60 Calories
1g fat
(Traditional sautéed mushrooms: 210
Calories, 22g fat)

I didn't think I would be able to produce acceptable "sautéed" mushrooms without butter or, at the very least, a bit of oil. I was wrong. These mushrooms are not only good—they are addictive. Use them as a garnish, stir them into soups and sauces, or eat them right out of the pan, if you are as wild about mushrooms as I am.

8 ounces mushrooms, cleaned and quartered
½ cup dry sherry or red wine
½ cup chicken or vegetable stock

1 or 2 dashes low-sodium soy sauce
Freshly ground pepper to taste

1. Put the mushrooms and liquid (including soy sauce) into a non-reactive, nonstick heavy frying pan. Stir to combine everything very well.

2. Simmer, stirring occasionally. First the mushrooms will release a good deal of extra liquid. Continue simmering, stirring occasionally, until the liquid is almost gone. Let the mushrooms "fry" gently in their own juices for a few moments. Do not let them scorch or stick. Season with pepper to taste and serve, or refrigerate or freeze for later use.

"SMOOTHED-OUT" DRAINED COTTAGE CHEESE

Cottage cheese is lumpy; that is one of the unfortunate facts of the gastronomic universe. But it can be smoothed out to form a very pleasing spread, dip, or recipe ingredient. "Smoothed out" drained cottage cheese—especially with herbs, spices, or crushed fruit blended in—is so good it's hard to stop eating it once you start.

1. Put very-low-fat cottage cheese (1 percent fat or less) in the blender. (In this case, the processor will not do. The resulting cheese would be grainy rather than smooth.) Blend, using a rubber spatula to push the cheese onto the blades as necessary, until perfectly smooth and creamy. If you wish, blend in fresh snipped chives, shredded sorrel, shredded mint, or—indeed—any fresh herbs you like. Very ripe crushed strawberries, peaches, or the like are also delicious when blended in.

2. Scrape the mixture into a cheesecloth-lined sieve over a bowl, and refrigerate for several hours or overnight. Use the unflavored "smoothed-out" drained cheese in recipes or as a compelling spread for toast and crackers. And, of course, the flavored "smoothed-out" cheese is great on bread, as a dip, or even straight out of the bowl.

"CREAM CHEESE"

You will lose approximately ¼ to ⅓ of the volume of yogurt or fromage blanc through draining.

This "cream cheese" is thick and creamy, perfect for spreading on bread or toast or dolloping onto baked potatoes in place of high-fat sour cream, cream cheese, or butter. Use it, too, as a base for "Mayonnaise" (following recipe) or creamy salad dressing. Yogurt cheese is very easy to make and so versatile that it pays to have some on hand in the refrigerator at all times. Draining fromage blanc results in a milder cheese than yogurt.

1. Line a sieve or colander with a long piece of damp doubled cheesecloth. (Rinse it first in cool water, then wring it out well.) Place the lined sieve over a large bowl. Dump in very-low-fat yogurt or fromage blanc, fold the cheesecloth over to cover well, and leave in

the refrigerator for 24 hours. Every once in a while, pour off the liquid that accumulates in the bowl.

2. At the end of the 24-hour period upwrap the cheese and scrape it into a bowl or crock. Refrigerate.

Note: Add any of the following ingredients to the cheese to produce a delicious spread: crushed garlic marinated in wine vinegar; chopped fresh chives; chopped fresh dill; shredded smoked fish; minced, mixed vegetables (radishes, celery, carrots, red and yellow peppers).

"MAYONNAISE"

♡   *Makes approximately ¾ cup*

Forget real mayonnaise, yummy though it may be. The wicked stuff is made from egg yolks and a whole lot of oil, with a little mustard and wine vinegar thrown in. Pure unadulterated fat, with no redeeming value whatsoever. Slim Cuisine "Mayonnaise" is low-fat and low Calorie. Use it in salad recipes or as a sandwich spread. (See pages 201–12 for more ideas.) You may feel as smug as you please as you eat your salad and sandwiches: real mayo has 99 Calories and 11g fat per tablespoon; this version only 7 Calories, and 0.03g fat.

½ cup yogurt cheese or drained fromage blanc or a combination (preceding recipe) 1 to 2 teaspoons Dijon mustard, or to taste	3 to 4 tablespoons buttermilk 1 to 2 tablespoons wine vinegar Salt and freshly ground pepper to taste

Whisk all the ingredients together, adding the buttermilk and vinegar gradually, tasting as you go, until a mayonnaiselike consistency is achieved, and until the flavor pleases you. Season to taste. Refrigerate overnight for flavors to blend.

Note: Add any one of the following ingredients to your mayonnaise, if desired: crushed garlic; chili powder, hot or mild; Hungarian paprika, hot or mild; curry spices; red pepper purée (see page 27); tomato paste; or chopped fresh herbs.

 ## STABILIZED YOGURT

Heat applied to yogurt causes it to curdle. Very-low-fat yogurt seems to be more prone to curdling than yogurt with higher fat levels. Cornstarch stabilizes the yogurt so that it can be used in soups and hot sauces, but even stabilized yogurt must be simmered only gently. Boiling will cause it to "break" or become grainy.

2 teaspoons cornstarch blended with 1 tablespoon water	2½ cups skim milk yogurt, at room temperature

1. Whisk together the cornstarch, water, and yogurt.
2. Place the mixture into a nonreactive heavy saucepan. Gently bring to a simmer, stirring. Simmer gently for 5 minutes, stirring often.

Baked Vegetables

Everyone knows that potatoes can be baked with delicious effect. But did you ever think of baking a whole head of garlic? (Yes, I said garlic.) Or a large sweet onion? It can be done, and the results will delight you, both for immediate eating and for use in thickening soups, stews, and sauces.

 ☆ ## BAKED GARLIC

When garlic bakes in the oven for an hour or so, it loses its strong assertiveness and becomes mellow, sweet, and vaguely nutlike. The texture changes too; the meat of each clove softens into a purée. The purée is excellent as a thickening agent for soups, sauces, and stews. It imparts body and a mysterious and gentle flavor boost without adding salt, fat, or excess Calories. The whole baked heads of garlic also make a dandy starter for a dinner party. Be sure to use the largest, firmest, freshest heads of garlic you can find for this procedure.

Whole heads of garlic | **Toasted rounds of bread**

1. Preheat oven to 375 F.

2. Remove the papery outer covering of the whole garlic heads, but do not separate the cloves or peel them. Place as many whole heads of garlic on a large square of aluminum foil (shiny side in) as there are people to be served. Fold up the foil so that the cloves are completely wrapped.

3. Bake in the preheated oven for approximately 1¼ hours, depending upon the size of garlic heads.

4. Serve each diner a head of garlic and some bread. Separate the cloves. Hold a clove over a piece of bread and squeeze. The garlic purée will pop out, like toothpaste from a tube.

MICROWAVE VERSION OF
♡ ☆ ◔ ◛　　 BAKED GARLIC

If you try to put a whole head of garlic into the microwave to bake, you will end up with something quite horrid. The cloves become tough, and the taste becomes acrid and revolting. There *is* a way, however, to achieve a melting, mellow, and sweetly delicious garlic purée in the microwave. Be *very careful* when you remove the plastic wrap. Follow the directions meticulously, or you may get scalded by the steam.

1. Remove the papery outer covering from 2 to 3 large, firm heads of garlic, but do not peel them. Separate the cloves. Scatter them, in one layer, in an 8-inch-square, 1- to 2-inch-deep glass baking dish. Pour in water to a depth of a little more than ½ inch. Cover *tightly* with microwave plastic wrap.

2. Microwave on high for 10 minutes. Carefully remove from the oven (do not remove or loosen plastic wrap) and let stand for 10 minutes.

3. With tongs peel away a corner of the plastic wrap on the side *away from you*, to allow steam to escape. Be very careful: The steam is hot, and you don't want to get burned. With the tongs, remove the plastic wrap.

4. When the garlic is cool enough to handle, remove the skins (they will slip right off). Drain the garlic and place in a bowl. Mash with a fork or a wooden pestle. If desired, push through a sieve to make a very fine purée.

 # GARLIC PURÉE

Keep a supply of this lovely stuff in the refrigerator and use it to liven up all kinds of dishes. Stir it into soups and stews by the spoonful; use it to thicken sauces; and spread it on bread (mixed with quark or *Slim Cuisine* "Cream Cheese," if you wish). Garlic popcorn—air-popped popcorn with a good dollop of garlic purée—makes a simple, unbelievably savory snack. No salt is needed; the garlic flavor is sufficient.

1. To make a batch of garlic purée for later use, let heads of Baked Garlic (page 23) cool, unwrapped, for at least 5 minutes.

2. Gently separate the cloves and squeeze each over a fine-meshed sieve, so that the softened garlic pops into the sieve.

3. With a wooden spatula or spoon, rub the garlic through the sieve into a small container or bowl.

4. Cover tightly with plastic wrap and refrigerate until the purée is needed.

Note: If you are in a hurry, you may skip the sieve. Simply squeeze the cloves, one by one, over a bowl. When they have all been squeezed, use a rubber spatula to push the purée into a neat mound, cover tightly with plastic wrap, and refrigerate until needed.

♡ ☆ ▣　　　　# BAKED ONIONS

A baked onion served whole, sprinkled with fresh pepper and lemon juice, makes a lovely vegetable accompaniment to a meal. It can also be puréed in a blender and used as garlic purée can be used: to thicken sauces, soups, and stews, and to give them a low-fat, low-Calorie, and low-salt flavor and texture boost.

Large Spanish onions

1. Preheat the oven to 425 F.
2. Put the onions on a double sheet of aluminum foil, shiny side out, but do not wrap them. Bake for 1¼ hours, or until very soft and almost collapsed.
3. With a sharp knife, cut off the stem and root ends of the onions. Remove and discard the blackened skin and first layer. Serve as they are with pepper and lemon juice, or put the onions into a blender and purée them for use in other recipes.

▣ *Note:* To prepare this in a microwave, wrap a large Spanish onion in microwave plastic wrap. Place a sheet of paper towels on the carousel. Put the wrapped onion on the towels. Microwave on high for 3 minutes, turn over, and microwave on high for an additional 3 minutes. Let stand for 1 or 2 minutes.

♡ BAKED OR GRILLED PEPPERS

Both yellow and red bell peppers (green peppers may be used too, but they are not as pretty, or as sweet) have an enticing fleshy sweetness. When baked or broiled the skin chars. Peel off the blackened skin and the meat of the pepper is revealed: jewel-bright, tender, and splendidly flavorful. The baked pepper can be cut into strips, sprinkled with wine vinegar, and served as a vegetable; or puréed and served as a sauce or a garnish. Delicious juices will accumulate in the baking pan as the peppers cook. More will accumulate in the container in which the peppers are stored. Save these juices for sauces and salad dressing.

1. Preheat oven to 425 F. Place peppers on a foil-lined sheet (shiny side out).

2. Bake for 1 to 1¼ hours, turning the peppers with tongs two or three times during baking. The skins will blacken and char.

3. Enclose the hot peppers in a paper bag and let stand for 10 minutes. Steam will form between the charred skin and the flesh, making peeling much easier.

4. With your fingers, strip off the charred skin and discard it. Discard the seeds and the stem. Refrigerate the peppers as they are, or purée them in a blender and refrigerate. The peppers will keep in the refrigerator for a week. The purée can be frozen.

Note: If you have a gas cooker, roast the peppers by placing them directly on the flame of the plate on the gas stove. As the peppers blacken and char, turn them with tongs. Or they may be cut in half and grilled, cut side down, until they blacken and char. When blackened and charred, continue with steps 3 and 4, as above. Both these methods are quicker than using the oven.

Roasted red peppers in brine are also available in jars from many supermarkets and specialty food shops.

♡ ☆   # BAKED EGGPLANT

The chopped flesh of a baked eggplant is a wonderful filler for hamburgers and meatballs. It adds moistness and lightness, and cuts the Calories without adding any taste of its own. Even if you hate eggplant, you will love what it does to ground meat. For a delicious Middle Eastern dip, try the baked flesh, puréed or mashed with baked garlic, baked onion, and roasted pepper purées, yogurt, chopped tomatoes, herbs and spices (cumin, coriander leaves, cayenne). Serve with pita bread triangles or crudités.

Whole eggplants

1. Preheat oven to 400 F.
2. Pierce the eggplants in several places with a fork or thin skewer. Bake directly on the oven rack for 30 to 40 minutes, until soft and collapsed. Let cool.
3. Cut away the stems, strip off and discard the skins, and chop finely or mash. (If the clumps of seeds are large and tough, they may be discarded.)

♡ ☆ ◷ ▬   # MICROWAVE VERSION OF BAKED EGGPLANT

Eggplants must be pierced before they are microwaved, or they may explode. To make eggplant purée to use as a filler that provides moistness in meatballs, hamburgers, and sausages, they must be steamed in ½ inch water. Again, be very careful not to scald yourself with the steam.

1. Place 1 eggplant (½ pound) in an 8-inch-square, 1- to 2-inch-deep glass baking dish. Pour in ½ inch water. Cover tightly with microwave plastic wrap. Microwave on high for 6 minutes. Remove from the oven but do not uncover. Let rest for 5 minutes.

2. With tongs, very carefully peel away one corner of the plastic wrap on the side away from you to allow steam to escape. It is very hot, so use caution: you do not want to scald your hands or face. With the tongs, remove plastic wrap. When the eggplant is cool enough to handle, strip off the skin with a dull knife. Chop the pulp very finely with a chef's knife.

BAKED TURNIPS, CARROTS, PARSNIPS, AND RUTABAGAS

♡ ☆ ❋

Why condemn turnips, carrots, parsnips, and rutabagas to a watery, vitamin-stripped death? Forget boiling. Bake them so that they steam in their own juices. Instead of poor flabby things, they will be tender and succulent with a deep, caramelized flavor. When mashed or puréed, these baked vegetables are very useful for thickening and giving body to soups and stews. They may also be eaten as they are, or mashed with a bit of buttermilk and Parmesan cheese. Or they may be baked into a crusty gratin (see page 174).

| Turnips | Carrots |
| Parsnips | Rutabagas |

1. Preheat the oven to 425 F.

2. Peel the turnips and rutabagas. Scrub the carrots and parsnips. Leave them unpeeled if they are to be eaten whole, peel them if they are to be mashed. Quarter the rutabagas.

3. Wrap the turnips loosely in aluminum foil, shiny side in. Crimp well so that no steam escapes. Do the same with the parsnips, carrots, and rutabagas. Bake for 1 to 1¼ hours, until tender.

INGREDIENTS

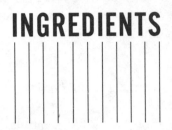

Stock

Stock is vital to Slim Cuisine. If your stock is high-quality, your food will be, too. Avoid bouillon cubes and powders that are laden with salt and monosodium glutamate.

♡ ☆ ❄ ## BASIC CHICKEN STOCK

This is very simple to make, but it does take time. The recipe can be multiplied and it freezes beautifully, so set aside a leisurely evening or slow Saturday to make a huge batch. Freeze it in small containers or in ice cube trays, and then pull out as needed. An easy way to make the stock is to keep simmering the chicken in the liquid for the full cooking time, until it completely falls apart. If you are using a whole chicken, do not succumb to this method. Yes, the stock will be very full-bodied, but the chicken will have cooked to rags and be good for nothing but the cat. Far better to remove the chicken when it is tender and succulent and can be used in any number of delicious dishes. Use the bones to finish the stock. Boiling hens are almost impossible to find these days, so a roasting chicken is what you will need for this recipe. For best results, use a free-range chicken. Of course, if you wish you may use just wings, necks, and backs, or even chicken carcasses that you have saved in the freezer. If you use these scraps, simmer them until they have given their all to the broth; there is no need to go through the cooling and boning process described in steps 2 and 3. Homemade stock, meticulously strained and skimmed, contains negligible Calories.

Makes about 2 quarts

One 2½- to 3½-pound dressed chicken, or chicken wings, backs, and necks
3 celery stalks
2 parsnips

2 carrots
1 small onion
1 garlic clove, unpeeled
Several sprigs parsley
Water

1. Wash the chicken well inside and out, and pull off excess fat. Scrub the celery, parsnips, and carrots, leaving the carrots and parsnips unpeeled. Peel the onion. Cut the celery, carrots, parsnips, and onion into chunks.
2. In a large pot of 5 quarts of water, boil the chicken and any extra chicken parts. After 10 minutes, skim all foam and scum from the top. Add the garlic, vegetables, and parsley. Reduce the heat so that the liquid stays at a steady simmer. Simmer, partially covered, until the chicken is tender and succulent, about 50 minutes to 1 hour. Let the chicken cool in the partially covered pot for at least 1 hour, but no more than 2 hours. If you are using backs, necks, wings, and carcasses, just let it simmer for another 30 minutes to 1 hour, and then proceed to step 4.
3. Carefully remove the whole chicken from the pot. (It will still be quite warm, so be careful.) Pull the chicken meat from the bones and tear it into chunks. Discard the skin and all bits of fat and gristle. Place the meat in a wide shallow container, moisten with a bit of the stock, cover well, and refrigerate immediately for use in a later recipe. Return all bones to the stock. Bring to a boil, reduce heat, and simmer, partially covered, for another 30 minutes.
4. Carefully strain it in batches through a fine sieve or strainer. Press down on the solids to extract all the juice and nutrients. Pour the stock into clean jars, cover tightly, and refrigerate overnight.

5. By the next day the fat will have risen to the top of each jar of stock and solidified. Meticulously scrape away every speck of fat and discard it. The stock itself may have jelled. Don't worry, this is just a sign that you have made a good, gelatin-rich broth. It will liquefy again when heated. Pour the defatted stock into containers and store in the freezer until needed.

CHICKEN WING STOCK

 Makes about 10 cups

This is a very easy-to-make and full-bodied stock, less expensive than the previous one. It is so rich that it jells when chilled. In my kitchen, my assistant, Sandie Perry, and I get double our money's worth out of chicken wings by using them twice. After we've drained the solids from a batch of stock, we pick out the wings, combine them with fresh vegetables and do the whole thing over again. As far as I'm concerned, chicken stock is the best sautéing medium there is. Make it regularly in large quantities, and freeze it in small batches (or in ice cube trays). Thaw (in the microwave, if you have one) when needed.

2½ to 3½ pounds chicken wings, plus backs, necks, and carcasses, if you have them	2 carrots
	1 small onion
	Water
3 celery stalks	A few cloves garlic, unpeeled
2 parsnips	Several sprigs parsley

    1. Wash the chicken pieces well. Scrub the celery, parsnips, and carrots, leaving the carrots and parsnips unpeeled. Peel the onion. Cut the celery, carrots, parsnips, and onion into chunks.

    2. In a large pot, boil the chicken parts in 4 quarts of water. After 10 minutes, skim all foam and scum from the top. Add the garlic, vegetables, and parsley. Reduce the heat so that the liquid stays at a steady simmer. Simmer, partially covered, for 2½ to 3 hours. Let cool slightly.

3. Carefully strain the stock through a fine sieve or strainer in batches. Press down on the solids to extract all the juice. Pour the stock into clean jars, cover tightly, and refrigerate overnight.

4. By the next day the fat will have risen to the top of each jar of stock and solidified. Meticulously scrape away every speck of fat and discard it. Pour the defatted stock into containers, label with the date, and store in the freezer until needed.

Simple Stock

I have racked my brains and ransacked the groceries, health-food, and gourmet shops for a quick substitute for homemade stock. Here are three thoughts for cooks in a hurry.

1. Most Chinese restaurants have huge quantities of good-quality chicken stock on hand. In many cases, salt and monosodium gluta-mate are not added until the moment the stock is transformed into a soup or added to a cooked dish. If you are a regular customer at a local restaurant, ask the owner if you can occasionally buy some. Often, if you bring a container, the proprietors of many such places (if they know you) will cheerfully fill it for a very modest price. When you get the stock home, it needs to be chilled so that the fat can be skimmed off. Quick-chill, if necessary, by placing the stock in the freezer for a few minutes or by dropping a few ice cubes into it.

2. There are vegetable stock cubes and vegetable bouillon pastes and powders available, but most of the ones I have tried taste perfectly awful and will ruin any recipe you add them to (as will chicken stock cubes). There are, however, a few palatable low-salt, low-fat vegetable bouillon powders available in some gourmet and health-food shops. There is also an excellent Swiss powder meant to be used to make a hot vegetable bouillon *drink*. It contains *no* salt or fat. If you use one of these powders to sauté, don't even bother to reconstitute them. Simply add water to your onions and garlic, then sprinkle in a little of the bouillon powder.

3. If you resort to a canned chicken stock, make sure it is a *low-sodium* one. It may not be as good (and as economical) as the home-made stuff, but it sure is a bonus for cooks in a hurry! Keep the cans

in the refrigerator, so that when you use it you can skim off and discard the congealed fat globules.

♡ ☆ ❄ # VEGETABLE STOCK

Vegetable stock is quicker and less expensive than chicken stock. There are many versions, one of which follows. Vegetable stock is a boon for vegetarians or for anyone who does not want a meaty stock. Again, as with chicken stock, make it in large quantities and freeze it in small containers or in ice cube trays.

4 leeks	4 parsnips
5 celery stalks with leaves	2 to 3 fresh bay leaves, or 1 dried
2 large onions	3 to 4 sprigs fresh thyme
4 ounces mushrooms	Handful of fresh parsley
4 white turnips	1 large potato
5 carrots	Freshly ground pepper to taste

1. Trim the vegetables and clean them well, but leave them unpeeled. Cut them into large chunks. Place them in a deep pot and cover generously with cold water. Bring to a boil.

2. Skim off foam. Partially cover pot, lower heat, and simmer for approximately 1 hour.

3. Season with some freshly ground pepper. Strain the broth in batches through a fine sieve or strainer (discard the solids). Cool and refrigerate. Use the stock within 3 days, or store in the freezer for later use.

Smoked Chicken

There are very good smoked chickens available in some supermarkets, specialty shops, and delicatessens. A smoked chicken is ready to eat, so it needs no further cooking other than a brief warming, but it's good cold too. It can be stored in the freezer for months, with no appreciable loss of quality. Use smoked chicken in sandwiches (for suggestions see page 213) or to give a wonderful smoky accent to pasta dishes (see page 159). If you can, freeze your smoked chicken in pieces, because you will only need a little bit at a time. Never throw away the smoked chicken bones and scraps. Save them in the freezer until you have enough to make stock. The stock will have a haunting and lovely smoky edge, making it perfect for split pea and bean soups, chestnut soup, some sauces—anywhere you want a smoky taste without resorting to high-fat smoked bacon, ham, and so on.

Dairy Products

Learn to read labels! Dairy products are an incomparable source of calcium, high-quality protein, and fat-soluble vitamins. Full-fat and part-skim products, however, have a distressingly high fat content, and have no place in the diet of *anyone* who cares about his or her health and weight control. Read the labels—bring a magnifying glass to the store with you if necessary—and buy dairy products that have a fat content of 1 percent or less (preferably less).

SKIM MILK YOGURT

Low-fat yogurt is an extremely valuable and useful product. Use it in place of sour cream and crème fraîche, or drain it to form a delightful "Cream Cheese" (see page 21). Yogurt cream cheese can be turned into a fat-free, low-Calorie "Mayonnaise" (see page 22).

Undrained skim milk yogurt can also be used in cooking in place of cream. If the yogurt is to be simmered in a sauce or cooked dish, it must be stabilized to prevent curdling (see page 23).

The Magic of Yogurt

Ilya Metchnikoff was obsessed with *Lactobacillus bulgaris*. Metchnikoff, a Nobel Laureate and the subdirector of the Pasteur Institute in Paris, believed the human aging process to be tragic and premature. He was convinced that a regular diet of yogurt (the result of this bacteria in milk) would significantly prolong life and hold senility and physical degeneration at bay. Secure in his belief, Metchnikoff wrote a book, *The Prolongation of Life*, and fed himself lavish amounts of yogurt until the end of his life. That end, alas, came at the age of seventy-one—a decent enough span, but not the century-plus length of years he was so sure he would achieve.

Today, almost seventy years after the publication of Metchnikoff's book, yogurt is a supermarket staple. Although it won't help you to live forever, it is a magnificent cooking ingredient—tangy, custardy, and smooth—and the low-fat version is one of the standbys of Slim Cuisine. Thank you, Monsieur Metchnikoff: How lovely it is to indulge in mayonnaise and creamy salad dressings without indulging in fat and excess Calories as well.

SKIM MILK BUTTERMILK

American buttermilk is delicious. It is not really *buttermilk*—that is, the liquid leftover from the butter-making process. It is, rather, a cultured product. Look for the kind cultured from skim milk. Skim milk buttermilk is thick, creamy, and only slightly tangy. The taste is very similar to that of sour cream. It gives a lovely flavor and texture to desserts and to low-fat "mayonnaise"-type salad dressings. It is worth searching for. Most large supermarkets carry buttermilk. If it is that ridiculous brand of buttermilk that has been cultured from skim milk but has flakes of butter (!) in it, strain before using. Strawberries, buttermilk, and a light sprinkling of brown sugar make a heavenly finish to a meal. Buttermilk is also an important component of Slim Cuisine ice creams (see pages 222–26).

PARMESAN CHEESE

A classic Italian grating cheese with an emphatic taste, a little bit of Parmesan goes a very long way. One tablespoon of this medium-fat cheese adds approximately 25 Calories (1.8g fat) to a recipe. If possible, buy real Italian Parmigiano Reggiano and grate it yourself as follows:

Cut the cheese into small chunks. Put them in the blender. Blend until finely grated. Store in the refrigerator or freezer. Save the rind; Parmesan rind is one of the magic ingredients of Slim Cuisine. Use a piece of it when simmering certain sauces, soups, and ragoûts. When the dish is finished, discard the rind. It will have imparted a good Parmesan flavor but very little in the way of Calories and fat.

MOZZARELLA CHEESE

Another Italian classic, this one melts into a bland, gooey, creamy, pully mass—quite wonderful. Buy real Italian or Italian-style mozzarella. It is medium-fat (part-skim), and may come packed in liquid.

LOW-FAT COTTAGE CHEESE

Buy *low-fat* (less than 1 percent) cottage cheese only. Smooth it out in the blender and drain it in a cheesecloth-lined sieve and you have a lovely, creamy substance perfect for spreading on bread and bagels and using in all kinds of recipes: Liptauer Cheese, Creamy Pesto, Strawberry Cream, Pasta Alfredo . . . Please note that a processor doesn't work here. Processing cottage cheese renders it grainy; blending, however, produces a heavenly smoothness. Throughout Canada, one can buy "pressed cottage cheese"—a smooth, creamy skim milk cottage cheese with no lumps, absolutely wonderful. What a shame that it is not available in the United States, but blending and draining the usual lumpy kind give superb results. In some parts of America, one can buy skim milk farmer's cheese, hoop cheese, baker's cheese, or pot cheese. All of these skim milk curd cheeses (nonlumpy as they are) are marvelous in Slim Cuisine recipes. If you are lucky enough to find them (*read the labels* to make sure the fat content is below 1 percent), by all means use them in recipes calling for "smoothed-out" drained cottage cheese.

QUARK

It's neither the cry of an inebriated duck nor (as a physics text might indicate) a subatomic particle. Quark is a German, creamy-smooth, soft, spreadable skim milk curd cheese. Quark is wonderful spread on bread or used in recipes in place of cream cheese, sour cream, or even whipped cream. I live in England now, where quark is available in many supermarkets, and I find it infinitely useful in luxurious low-fat cooking. I am absolutely delighted to learn that an excellent domestic American quark is now available, as of this writing, in at least sixteen states. It has been spotted by my foodie spies in gourmet-food stores in New York, Atlanta, Georgia, and other places.

FROMAGE BLANC

Fromage blanc (sometimes called fromage frais) is another absolutely invaluable European dairy product. Fromage blanc can be made entirely of skim milk, and so can be entirely fat-free. Although it is called fromage—cheese—it is not particularly cheeselike; it is more like sour cream or crème fraîche in taste and texture. What delight for hedonistic practitioners of low-fat cooking. Like quark, low-fat fromage blanc, produced by local independent dairies, is now available in some American supermarkets and specialty food shops.

Seasonings

GARLIC

Garlic is an important part of Slim Cuisine and adds a wonderful depth of flavor and richness to many preparations. Slim Cuisine cooking techniques involve steaming, poaching, baking, simmering, and boiling; no frying or sautéing in oils or fats. It is these latter techniques that bring out garlic's overpowering qualities. On the other hand, in salads and dressings that call for raw garlic, the taste of garlic will be stronger. By all means in those recipes leave out the garlic if you wish.

When shopping, choose garlic carefully. Lift the bulbs and squeeze them. They should be heavy and firm. Never buy heads that have shriveled or bruised cloves. (Remember, a clove is one section, a bulb or head is the whole thing.) And never buy garlic that is visibly sprouting. If, when peeling and mincing the cloves, you find that each contains a greenish sprout in the center, split the clove, remove the sprout, and discard it. Store garlic bulbs in a cool, well-ventilated part of the kitchen. They should not be tightly wrapped—a basket is the ideal receptacle. Never refrigerate them. Do *not* use garlic salt, garlic powder, or other processed garlic products. They will impart a harsh, rancid, and unpleasant taste to your cooking.

When crushing garlic use a mallet, not a garlic press. The press is an infamous utensil that releases all of garlic's strong, indigestible qualities. The mallet is handy for peeling the cloves as well as crushing them. Hit the clove with the mallet, remove the loosened skin, and proceed.

GINGER

Fresh ginger has become a supermarket staple. Once you try it, you will be delighted with its clean, bracing flavor. Always peel it first with a paring knife or a swivel-bladed peeler, and then grate or mince it.

BLACK PEPPER

Use whole peppercorns cracked in a peppermill, as needed, instead of packaged preground pepper. The taste it imparts to your recipes will be flavorful, not merely sharp. White peppercorns are the same berry as the black ones, at a different stage of ripeness. White pepper is the mature berry with the outer husk removed. Black pepper is slightly underripe. If you dislike black specks in your food, keep a mill filled with white peppercorns for light-colored food.

SALT

Somehow we have become accustomed to large quantities of salt in our food. Try cutting down gradually and learn to savor the taste of good, fresh ingredients without their usual cloak of saltiness. Salt is invaluable as a flavor enhancer, and a sprinkle here and there brings out natural flavors in a wonderful way. For reasons of good health and good taste, wean yourself from the excess-salt habit. The instructions in recipes in this book specify "salt to taste." Try to make it a sprinkle, not an avalanche.

Canned beans (chick-peas, kidney beans, pinto and cannelini beans, et cetera) are excellent staples, as is canned tuna, but they contain large amounts of salt. Wash most of the salt away by emptying the contents of the can into a colander and then rinsing well under cold water.

SOY AND TERIYAKI SAUCES

These two excellent Chinese condiments are very useful with mushrooms. Buy low-sodium soy and teriyaki sauces only. Simmer the fungi in a mixture of stock and wine, with a dash of soy sauce or teriyaki sauce, and you won't miss the butter or oil.

SUGAR

Like salt, sugar is very much a matter of taste. And, like salt, sugar is an amazingly good flavor enhancer. It helps bring out natural flavors and put them into balance. Unfortunately, most people do not think of sugar as another seasoning. They think of the sweet stuff as a major ingredient, and consume an enormous amount of it each day. The goal should not be to experience an overwhelming sweetness, but to experience sweetness in concert with other flavors. Learn to orchestrate ingredients, and to use them with finesse, so that the overall effect is harmonious. Sugar is just one part of the orchestra; fight the urge to make it a soloist.

CHILI PEPPERS

Fresh chiles have found their way into the supermarkets, and welcome they are to lovers of incendiary cuisine. There are thousands of kinds of chili peppers in the world; out of the profusion only a few find their way here. You will need to experiment with what your local market has to offer, but if you love edible fire, as I do, you will find such experimentation pure pleasure. Fresh chiles can be searingly hot; exercise caution when working with them. Always wash and trim them under cold running water. If your skin is sensitive, or if you have a cut on your hand, wear rubber gloves. If you don't use gloves, wash your hands very well with soap and water before rubbing your eyes, cuddling your sweetie, or hugging the baby. Two kinds of canned chiles are convenient to have on hand: green chiles (fairly mild) and jalapeños (very hot). Look for them in the Mexican-style foods section of the supermarket or gourmet shop.

TOMATOES

At certain times of the year, there are no tomatoes in the shops, only a bewildering array of pulpy, pale-pink, tennis ball–like impostors. Tomato lovers treat these objects with the scorn they deserve and depend upon canned Italian tomatoes until summer comes along, bringing its ripe bursting-with-flavor, ruby beauties. In the winter, if you long for fresh tomatoes, keep store-bought tomatoes at room temperature, in a closed paper bag. In a few days to a week they will have ripened and may even taste vaguely like tomatoes, although not like full-fledged summer beauties. To peel a fresh tomato, immerse it in boiling water for 10 seconds, then cut out the stem and slip off the skin. The seeds may be removed with your finger. Or, if you have a gas stove, spear a tomato on a long fork and hold it right over the gas flame until the skin splits (a few seconds is all it takes). Then strip off the skin. Tomato skins and seeds pass right through the human digestive system untouched, so you won't be losing valuable nutrients. If canned tomatoes seem particularly acidic, add a pinch of sugar when you cook them.

SUN-DRIED TOMATOES

The word was that sun-dried tomatoes were the ketchup of the eighties. In the United States, they began as something trendy or faddish, but—as do all versatile, excellent, and delicious foodstuffs—they have settled into the well-deserved role of useful staple. How I love the leathery, intensely flavored things! Sun-dried tomatoes are available dry pack (no oil) in cellophane bags or in bulk, and also minced in jars. Since the classic problem of nonfat cooking is lack of flavor, a foodstuff like sun-dried tomatoes, which contributes a wonderful wallop of nonfat flavor, is pure pleasure. American sun-dried tomatoes are less salty than Italian ones. I have seen dry-pack sun-dried tomatoes in some supermarkets across the country, and in countless specialty and gourmet shops. Use them in sauces, soups, and stews. Such dishes simmer for a while; therefore, the tomatoes need no reconstituting in advance.

HERBS

Fresh herbs bring a dimension of freshness and clear flavor that is never realized with the dried variety. A good rule of thumb: Use three times the amount of fresh herbs as dried. Do taste as you go, though, and be flexible. Be especially careful of dried herbs. Too much of a dried herb will give unpleasant results. And watch the quality of your dried herbs. They become old and musty all too easily. Buy them in small amounts and store them, tightly covered, in a cool, dark place. (A shelf above the stove is the *worst* possible place!) To release the flavor components in dried herbs, crumble them between your fingers as you scatter them into the pot.

SPICES

Spices are a collection of aromatic barks, seeds, roots, and buds that are used to season food. Buy them in small quantities, store them, tightly covered, in a cool, dark place, and try not to keep them beyond six months. When their oils turn rancid, they are unusable. Through kitchen experiment, learn the tastes of various spices, and learn the way they harmonize or clash with other spices and with various food-stuffs. Soon you will be seasoning food to please your own palate.

WINE

Dry red and white wine, dry sherry, and dry vermouth are important Slim Cuisine ingredients. If you cook the wine *briskly*—that is, boil it until there is just about no liquid left—then you don't need to worry about the alcohol (and the alcohol Calories) in such wines. As they boil down, the alcohol evaporates. You are left with an intense and delicious flavor, but it won't make anyone drunk, and it won't cause anyone to consume empty alcohol Calories. Flaming the alcohol, or gently simmering it, does not eliminate all the alcohol, so do make sure that you boil it right down. There is no need to invest in vintage wines for your cooking, but don't use a wine you wouldn't drink on its own.

BALSAMIC VINEGAR

This is another Italian ingredient that originally caught on in the United States as a gourmet fad, but has settled into a classic staple. Balsamic vinegar is produced by boiling the must of Trebbiano di Spagna grapes until it thickens and caramelizes, then culturing it in wooden barrels. The flavor, intensity, color, and quality of the finished product are a result of the type of wood, the size of the barrel, and the length of time the liquid is cured. The finished balsamic vinegar— the *real* stuff—is very expensive. Most of the balsamic vinegar you will find in supermarkets and gourmet shops is much more affordable and is not the real stuff—it is factory-made rather than cottage-produced in the traditional wood-cask manner—but still, it is *so good*. It makes a superb salad dressing or a sauce for steamed vegetables, potatoes, fish, or chicken breasts. I have an elegant little pocket flask I keep filled with balsamic vinegar, so that in restaurants I can dress my salad myself, with panache.

EQUIPMENT

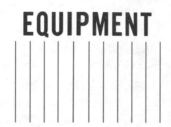

Nonreactive Cookware

Cast-iron, tin, and aluminum cookware will react with acid ingredients such as tomatoes, wine, and citrus juices to produce off flavors and discolorations. To avoid these problems, use nonreactive cookware, such as enameled cast iron, stainless steel, flameproof glass and ceramic, and nonstick coatings. Because no added fat is used in Slim Cuisine, you will find the nonstick cookware invaluable. When choosing such equipment, go for weight. Hefty, heavy-bottomed pots and pans cook evenly and will ensure success. Read the directions that come with your cookware. Many nonstick pots and pans must be seasoned, sometimes by rubbing the nonstick finish with oil, sometimes by simmering milk in the pan. If the instructions specify oil, spray the pan liberally with nonstick cooking spray instead, and smear it around with a paper towel. You should have to do this only once, when the pan is brand-new.

An enameled cast-iron frying pan is handy for sautéing—for those times when you want a nonreactive pot, but not a nonstick one (see Sautéed Onions, page 15). If you plan to do a lot of stir-frying (easy to do without fat, see page 14), you might want to invest in a wok. Big ones with a cover, steamer rack, and nonstick interior are available in cookware departments throughout the country. They work with both gas and electric stoves.

A steamer is an absolute necessity for vegetables. It can be used for fish, chicken breasts, and rice as well. Buy a folding one that fits into a large saucepan or, better still, a stockpot with a perforated steamer-basket that fits inside. If necessary, improvise a steamer with a colander set in a saucepan. If you live near a Chinese market, consider acquiring a Chinese bamboo steamer that fits in a wok. Such a steamer is fairly inexpensive, easy and versatile to use, and attractive.

For straining, puréeing, and draining yogurt and fromage blanc, have several nonreactive sieves or strainers on hand. Nylon-mesh sieves are perfect. Cheesecloth is essential to line the sieve when you use it to make "Cream Cheese" (see page 21). If you want to make fat-free ice creams, purées, dips, and so on, both a food processor and a blender are invaluable tools. You will use them again and again. A microwave oven, of course, makes a busy cook's life so much easier. And don't forget an assortment of wooden spoons and wire whisks standing in a jar by your work area, and a faithful set of measuring utensils, both spoons and cups.

MENU PLANNING

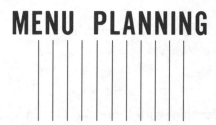

Preparing food the Slim Cuisine way means learning some new techniques and habits. It takes no longer to prepare and cook this way than any other kind of everyday cooking, if you plan ahead. Always keep a supply of baked eggplant and baked garlic purées in the refrigerator, for instance. Then, if you want to make meatballs or pesto, you don't have to bake the eggplant and garlic first before getting down to the business of the recipe itself. And Slim Cuisine ice cream is the fastest dessert imaginable, if the freezer is well stocked with frozen fruit and berries. You must keep low-sodium canned bouillon or a good stock powder, and drained yogurt and/or drained fromage blanc, on board as well.

DINNER PARTIES

All too often, dinner parties are excuses for total culinary depravity: creamed sauces, roasts with thick layers of fat, rich gravies, vegetables swimming in butter or olive oil, sugary desserts drowning in oceans of heavy cream and monstrous dollops of buttercream. It is almost as if the hostess/cook says: "The Robinsons are coming to dinner. Let's *kill* them!" As a devotee of Slim Cuisine, you know that culinary mayhem is obsolete, even at dinner parties. It is possible to entertain lavishly and deliciously without Calorie and fat overkill. Here are a few suggestions:

Turkey and Melon with Creamy Mint Pesto	64
Wild Mushroom Soup	80
Stuffed Flank Steak	123
Potato Gratin	192
Stir-"Fried" Zucchini with Lime and Cumin	175
Mango Sorbet	224
Mushroom Ravioli with Pepper Sauce	58, 161
Jellied Gazpacho	85
Broiled Fish Fillets with Mustard	91
Braised Fennel	183
Steamed Broccoli	182
Blackberry Gratin	228
Steamed Asparagus in Yellow Pepper Sauce	177, 133
Pork Medallions Esterhazy	124
Roast Potatoes with Roasted Garlic and Onion	195
Strawberries on Red and White Sauce	230
Poached Mushrooms Stuffed with Mint Raita and Beet Purée	57, 203, 181
Soup of Baked Vegetables	78
Steak with Garlic-Wine Sauce	122
Stir-"Fried" Cauliflower	177
Stuffed Potatoes	190
Blueberry Ice Cream	226
Kathleen Edwards's Tuna Mousse	62
Onion Soup	77
Chicken with Yellow Pepper Sauce	133
Creamed Spinach	180

Potato Cases Filled with Mushroom Ragoût   191, 185
Jellied Tropical Fruit   234

Shashi's Parma Aloo on a Bed of Mint Raita   68, 203
Turnip Soup   72
Lemon-Roasted Chicken   146
Onion-Tomato Relish   210
Stir-"Fried" Yellow and Red Peppers   179
Mixed Berries on Raspberry Sauce with Slim   229, 227
  "Whipped Cream"

Beet Purée in Endive Leaves   181
Cod en Papillote   94
Steamed Cauliflower with Red Pepper Sauce   161
Potato-Mushroom Gratin   192
Pineapple Sorbet with Black Currant Sauce   224, 229

Orange-Watercress Salad   204
Red Pepper Soup   75
Chicken Lasagna   159
Stir-"Fried" Asparagus   178
Almond Curd with Black Currant Sauce   234

Chilled Corn Soup   84
Penne with Pesto and Smoked Chicken   164
Fennel-Pepper Salad   207
Tomato-Basil Salad   204
Pineapple Sorbet   224

VEGETARIAN DINNER PARTIES

Liptauer Cheese   60
Wild Mushroom Soup   80
Pasta with Herbed Eggplant Sauce   168

| Green Salad with Slim Cuisine Dressing | 201 |
| Banana Ice Cream with Raspberry Sauce | 222, 229 |

Celeriac Rémoulade	66
Bean Soup	73
Grilled Vegetable Lasagna	150
Tomato-Basil Salad	204
Berries with Mango Sauce	230

ETHNIC FEASTS

For a wonderful dinner party, try a buffet of ethnic delicacies. The ethnic recipes in Slim Cuisine are all based on authentic ones, but they have been redesigned to eliminate fat. Even though the identifying fat of a particular cuisine is gone (lard for Mexico, olive oil for Italy, et cetera), the remaining flavor principles are unchanged.

MEXICAN

Salsa with Tortilla Chips	188, 218
Frijol-Albondiga Casserole	101
Chilaquiles	145
Stir-"Fried" Zucchini with Lime and Cumin	175
Mango Sorbet	224

ITALIAN

Tomato-Mozzarella Salad	204
Italian Sausage Balls served with Tomato Sauce and a dollop of Creamy Pesto surrounded by: Stir-"Fried" Peppers and Browned Onions	105, 166, 160, 179, 16
Sweet-and-Sour Zucchini	176
Braised Fennel	183
Fresh Berry Gratin	228

VEGETARIAN ITALIAN

| Tomato-Mozzarella Salad | 204 |
| Pasta Quills Tossed in Creamy Pesto | 160 |

EVERYDAY AND FAMILY MEALS

Everyday cooking needn't be elaborate; in fact, it shouldn't be. A hearty main dish and perhaps a salad or a vegetable and a good dessert should be more than enough. I'm particularly fond of family-type dishes that fill the house with heavenly aromas as they bubble happily away in the oven or on the stove.

Italian Sausage Soup	83
Tomato-Basil Salad	204
Strawberry Ice Cream	223
Shepherd's Pie	108
Creamed Spinach or	180
Corn Salad	208
Crunchy Bananas on Red and White Sauce	231
Carrot Soup	74
Baked Potatoes with a Choice of Fillings	185
Raspberry Ice Cream	223
Hamburgers with Browned Onions and Red Pepper Ketchup	107, 16, 167
Chinese Cabbage Salad	209
Apple Ice Cream	224
Oven-"Fried" Fish	92
French-"Fried" Potatoes	194
Rémoulade Sauce or Red Pepper Ketchup	66, 167
Selected Greens with Slim Cuisine Dressing	201
Banana Ice Cream	222

VEGETARIAN FAMILY MEALS

Pasta with Tomato Sauce	166
Garlic Bread (French or Italian bread spread with Garlic Spread)	216
Blueberry Ice Cream	226

Rajmaa	153
Tabouli	210
Blackberry Gratin	228

QUICK MEALS

For those who work full-time and then come home to cook, weekday meals must be quick. There are a wealth of quick, delicious, and deeply satisfying dishes to choose from. It seems a shame to have to succumb to the lure of high-fat, high-salt low-taste packaged and frozen foods because of limited time. Try the following suggestions, or make your own prepared meals by freezing small portions of Chili con Carne, Beef in Red Wine, Shepherd's Pie, Italian Meat Sauce, Chicken Lasagne, et cetera to be microwaved when needed.

Steak and Onions	122
Steamed Broccoli	182
Strawberry-Orange Ice Cream	224
Pizza	217
Italian Sweet-and-Sour Zucchini	176
Pineapple Sorbet	224
Fish Fillet en Papillote	94
Steamed New Potatoes	
Fresh Berry Gratin	228
Spaghetti with Italian Meat Sauce	114
Whole Wheat Toast and Garlic Spread	216
Strawberries with Raspberry Sauce	229

VEGETARIAN QUICK MEALS

Pasta with Helen's Terracotta Sauce	162
Steamed Cauliflower	

Apple Ice Cream   224

Farmer's Omelette   152
Beets (use cooked beets from the   189
    store) in Mustard Cream
Sliced Bananas or Peaches with a
    Yogurt or Fromage Blanc and
    Sprinkle of Brown Sugar

Pasta Shells Alfredo   156
Poached Mushroom Caps (unfilled)   57
Raspberry Ice Cream   223

II

Recipes

STARTERS

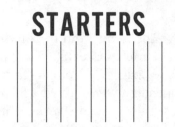

Starters should tease the palate, amuse the eyes, and launch the diner into the adventure of a meal. Serve a nibble or two with sherry or sparkling water in the living room, or serve a beautifully arranged first course at the dining table, but don't overwhelm the diner with an embarrassment of riches or the rest of the meal will be an anticlimax. Many of these starters would work well on a buffet table.

STUFFED POACHED MUSHROOMS

This is an absolutely beautiful way to begin a meal or to augment a buffet table. Choose mushrooms large enough to hold a filling but small enough to be picked up easily and popped into the mouth. These may be prepared 1 hour ahead of time, if desired.

Firm, white, medium or button
  mushrooms
About 3 ounces vegetable stock

About 3 ounces dry white
  vermouth
1 or 2 dashes soy sauce

FILLINGS:

The best, from both a visual and a taste point of view, are ♡ ☆ Beet Purée (page 181) and ♡ Mint Raita (page 203). But try these also: Creamy

Pesto, page 160; ♡ Tzatziki, page 63; Tonnato Sauce, page 65; ♡ Liptauer Cheese, page 60; ♡ ☆ Creamy Herb Dressing, page 202; ♡ ◔ ❄ Duxelles Cream, page 188; ♡ Mustard Cream, page 189.

1. Carefully remove the stems from the mushroom caps. Save the stems for another use (Duxelles Cream, for instance, see page 188, or Sautéed Mushrooms, see page 20). With a teaspoon, gently even out the mushroom cap opening so it will hold a filling nicely.

2. Pour the stock, vermouth, and soy sauce into a nonstick frying pan that will hold the mushroom caps in one layer. Bring the liquid to a boil. Add the mushroom caps, stem side up, reduce heat, cover, and simmer for 2 to 3 minutes. Uncover, raise heat, and cook, tossing the mushrooms in the pan for a minute or so, until the caps are cooked but still quite firm and the liquid is reduced and syrupy. Remove from the pan and drain upside down on paper towels.

3. With a teaspoon, neatly fill each cap with a filling of your choice. Use several different fillings of contrasting colors and textures for dramatic effect. Arrange on a serving platter.

MUSHROOM RAVIOLI

Makes 50 ravioli

Won ton wrappers (squares of noodle dough) are available in Chinese groceries. These delicate, mushroom-stuffed triangles are very special. Do not overwhelm them with sauce or the intense mushroom taste will not come through.

Flour
2 packages won ton wrappers
   (about 50 wrappers) (see note)
2½ cups Duxelles (page 187)
Fresh washed spinach or lettuce
   leaves

Tomato Sauce (page 166) or
   Yellow or Red Pepper Sauce
   (page 161)

1. Sprinkle your work surface with flour. Have 2 clean dishtowels at hand. Have a small bowl filled with water on your work surface.

2. Put 1 won ton wrapper flat on the work surface (keep the remainder covered with a clean dishtowel). Place 1 teaspoon Duxelles in the center of the wrapper. Dip your finger in the water and moisten the edge of the wrapper all around. Fold over to form a triangle and press the edges together so they adhere. Put the wrapper on the floured surface and cover with the second clean dishtowel. Repeat until all the wrappers and Duxelles are used up. (The ravioli may be frozen at this point: Dust 2 baking sheets with flour. Place the ravioli on the sheets in one layer, cover with plastic wrap, and freeze. When they are frozen solid, put them in a plastic bag and store in the freezer until needed. Do not thaw before cooking.)

3. Bring water to a boil in the bottom of a steamer. Line the steamer basket with spinach or lettuce leaves. Place the ravioli in one layer, on the greens. You will need to do this in several batches. Steam, covered, for 6 to 8 minutes, until tender. If steaming from frozen, steam for 10 to 12 minutes. Serve with Tomato Sauce or Yellow or Red Pepper Sauce. Ladle a bit of sauce over each serving, but do not overdo it.

Note: One package of egg roll wrappers may be used, if you can't find won ton wrappers. Cut each egg roll wrapper into quarters before proceeding with the recipe.

LIPTAUER CHEESE

Makes 1¼ cups

Conventionally, this Hungarian cheese spread is made with full-fat cheese and sour cream. My version has approximately one-third the Calories of the original, yet there is virtually no difference in taste.

1 pound skim milk quark or "smoothed out" drained cottage cheese
3 fluid ounces buttermilk
1 tablespoon sweet Hungarian paprika or paprika paste (see note)

Salt and freshly ground pepper to taste
2 teaspoons caraway seeds
Several dashes Tabasco sauce
1 teaspoon chopped capers

1. Combine all ingredients in a bowl and beat to a smooth paste.
2. Scrape the mixture into a colander lined with damp cheesecloth and let drain overnight.
3. Serve with pumpernickel bread or slices of cucumber and zucchini, or spread the mixture on bread or vegetable slices.

Hint: You can also mound the mixture into halved seeded and ribbed red, yellow, green, or purple peppers. Or serve this with crudités for dipping (try cauliflower, broccoli, zucchini, cucumber, fennel, carrot, turnip, radishes, et cetera).

You can vary this recipe with different ingredients. Try roasted garlic purée and chopped chives; finely chopped mushrooms simmered in stock until tender and dry, seasoned with a touch of nutmeg and cayenne pepper; puréed roasted red pepper with a squeeze of lemon juice.... The possibilities are endless!

Note: In Hungary, paprika paste (pure, puréed paprika) in tubes is available in every grocery or supermarket. I bought 2 dozen tubes the first time I saw them in Budapest. I am delighted to say that I have spotted the tubes in a few American gourmet shops. If you find them, buy several; the paste is incomparable in recipes such as this. The tubes with white caps are mild, those with red ones, fiery hot. If you can't find the paste, use real Hungarian rose paprika—mild, medium, or hot, according to your taste.

SMOKED FISH PÂTÉ

Makes 2 cups

A friend of mine, unused to cooking, made this for a buffet and the murmur went round, "Have you tasted the fish pâté? It's fabulous!" This is a great people pleaser.

6 to 8 ounces smoked trout or
  mackerel fillets, flaked
1 cup yogurt or fromage blanc
  "Cream Cheese" (page 21) or
  quark

2 tablespoons chopped fresh
  chives

1. Combine all ingredients in the bowl of a food processor.
2. Process until very smooth. Scrape into a crock and refrigerate overnight for the flavors to blend.
3. Serve with thin slices of whole wheat bread, toasted or not, as you prefer.

DILLED SMOKED SALMON SALAD

Makes 1½ cups

This tastes exactly as if it were made with crème fraîche. If you wish, pack it into a fish-shaped mold and refrigerate overnight. The next day, unmold it onto a sea of greens.

2 tablespoons drained yogurt
2 tablespoons buttermilk
¾ cup skim milk quark or
  "smoothed-out" drained
  cottage cheese

½ cup chopped fresh parsley
4 tablespoons chopped fresh dill
8 ounces smoked salmon,
  shredded
Freshly ground pepper to taste

1. Combine yogurt, buttermilk, and quark or cottage cheese in the bowl of a food processor and blend until smooth.
2. Stir in remaining ingredients.
3. Scrape the mixture into a crock and refrigerate overnight for flavors to blend.
4. Serve with endive and radicchio leaves. Each diner spoons a bit of the mixture into a leaf.

KATHLEEN EDWARDS'S TUNA MOUSSE

Serves 8

This creamy mousse is attractive in a fish-shaped mold. Decorate it beautifully for a buffet table.

3 teaspoons gelatin
2 tablespoons white wine vinegar
1¼ cups boiling chicken or
  vegetable stock
½ small onion, finely chopped
1 clove garlic
¼ teaspoon dried tarragon
Salt and freshly ground pepper to
  taste

8 ounces tuna packed in water,
  very well drained
4 tablespoons fromage blanc or
  yogurt
Cucumber, parsley, watercress,
  fresh tarragon, et cetera, as
  desired, for garnish

1. Place gelatin and vinegar in a blender or food processor and let stand for 1 minute.
2. Add the chicken or vegetable stock and blend.

3. Add all the remaining ingredients, except the fromage blanc or yogurt and garnish. Blend until perfectly smooth, about 1 minute.

4. Pour the tuna mixture into a bowl and let sit at room temperature until thickened but not set.

5. Stir the fromage blanc or yogurt into the tuna mixture. Pour into a mold and refrigerate until set.

6. To serve, unmold onto a serving plate and decorate with your choice of garnish. Serve with Melba toast or matzoh crackers, if you wish.

TZATZIKI

♡
Makes about 2 cups as a dip;
3 cups as a sauce

15 Calories per tablespoon
0.1g fat
(Traditional tzatziki: 30 Calories per
tablespoon, 2g fat)

Serve this zesty Greek mixture as a dip with toasted pita bread triangles, or as a sauce for steamed or broiled fish or lean meat (see Flank Steak, page 119). The meat juices mingling with the cold tzatziki are absolutely delicious.

4 cups skim milk yogurt	2 large cloves garlic, minced
2 large cucumbers	1½ teaspoons white wine vinegar
Salt	Freshly ground pepper to taste

1. Drain the yogurt for 24 hours (as described on page 21) if you want to serve the tzatziki as a dip. To serve it as a sauce, drain it for 6 to 7 hours only.

2. Peel the cucumbers. Cut them in half lengthwise. Use a teaspoon to scrape out the seeds, and discard them. Grate the cucumbers into a colander, salt them, and allow to drain for 30 minutes. This draws out their bitterness.

3. Place the minced garlic and vinegar in a small bowl and allow to marinate while the cucumbers are draining.

4. Rinse the drained cucumbers, squeeze them as dry as possible, and blot them on paper towels. Place them in the bowl with the marinated garlic. Add the drained yogurt and a few grindings of fresh pepper and stir. Serve at once, or store in the refrigerator. It will keep for several days and improve in flavor each day.

TURKEY AND MELON WITH CREAMY MINT PESTO

This is a colorful starter, and the combination of tastes and textures is unusual and pleasing. The plates may be arranged an hour or so before serving. The pesto may be made days in advance.

Ripe melon	Creamy Pesto (page 160) made
Thinly sliced smoked turkey	with fresh mint leaves
breast	Fresh mint leaves for garnish

1. Thinly slice the melon. Cut off the rind, and wrap each slice in a slice of turkey breast.

2. Arrange 3 wrapped slices on each plate. Place a dollop of pesto on the base of the plate. Garnish with fresh mint leaves and serve.

TONNATO SAUCE

♡

Makes 2 cups

25 Calories per tablespoon
0.1g fat
(Traditional tonnato sauce: 73 Calories
per tablespoon, 2.6g fat)

Tonnato is an Italian tuna mayonnaise, and one of my favorite cold sauces. It is traditionally served on slices of roasted veal or turkey breast. It is good as a dip for lightly steamed, chilled vegetables. It is also heavenly spread on toast.

1¼ cups yogurt or fromage blanc
  "Cream Cheese" (page 21)
Purée from 1 head baked garlic
  (page 23)
Two 7-ounce cans tuna packed in
  water, very well drained

Juice of ½ lemon
2 teaspoons capers
Salt and freshly ground pepper to
  taste

Combine all the ingredients in the container of a food processor and process until very smooth. Scrape into a bowl and refrigerate for at least 1 day. (The sauce will keep for a week and improve in flavor each day.) Serve as a dip with crudités or lightly steamed vegetables.

RÉMOULADE SAUCE

Makes about 4 cups

This sauce is versatile as a dip, sandwich spread, or sauce for julienned celeriac, cold poached chicken, steamed shrimp, or very lean, rare cold beef.

4 cups "Mayonnaise" made from yogurt or fromage blanc or a mixture of both (page 22)
2 teaspoons Dijon mustard
4 tablespoons capers, rinsed
4 tablespoons chopped cornichons (small sour gherkins)
4 tablespoons chopped fresh parsley

1 teaspoon paprika or paprika paste
6 scallions (green and white parts), chopped
Few drops Tabasco sauce
1½ teaspoon dried tarragon, crumbled

Combine all the ingredients with a wire whisk. Allow to ripen in the refrigerator for at least 1 hour before using.

HUMMUS

Makes 2½ cups

23 Calories per tablespoon
0.4g fat
(Traditional hummus: 48 Calories per tablespoon, 1.4g fat)

This is a low-fat version of a classic Middle Eastern chick-pea spread. The texture is rich and unctuous.

1½ tablespoons sesame seeds
Two 15½-ounce cans chick-peas, drained (reserve one-fourth to one-third of the liquid from 1 can)

Purée from 1 head baked garlic (page 23)
Juice of 2 large lemons

1. Toast the sesame seeds in a small heavy frying pan. Stir them constantly and do not allow them to scorch.

2. Place the sesame seeds in a blender or food processor and process until they are pulverized.

3. Add all the remaining ingredients, including the reserved chick-pea liquid. Process until very smooth and creamy; it should have the consistency of mashed potatoes. Add a little more of the chick-pea liquid if the mixture is too thick, and add a bit more lemon juice if you prefer a sharper taste. Serve as a sandwich spread or a dip with toasted pita bread wedges and raw vegetables.

Variations:

1. Mix hummus with an equal amount of quark or "smoothed-out" drained cottage cheese and use it as a filling for baked potatoes or potato cases (see page 191).

2. Thin with chicken or vegetable stock to a saucelike consistency, and toss with hot pasta.

ALOO CHAT

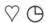

Makes 4 cups

Potatoes, coriander, and chili make up my favorite Indian starter. It is sour, spicy, and stimulating.

2 small, fresh green chiles, stemmed, seeded, and minced	4 tablespoons thinly sliced scallions
8 medium new potatoes, steamed until tender and diced	Salt to taste
4 tablespoons coarsely chopped fresh coriander	4 tablespoons fresh lemon juice

Gently toss all ingredients together. Allow to sit at room temperature for at least 30 minutes before serving.

SHASHI'S PARMA ALOO (STUFFED POTATOES, INDIAN STYLE)

Makes 8 pieces

This glorious dish is an old family recipe of Shashi Rattan's. I have omitted the oil and substituted lemon juice for hard-to-find mango powder. As the potatoes bake, the spicy coating blackens in places and forms a delicious crust. Parma Aloo are good served hot or cold. I think they taste best eaten with the fingers.

½ teaspoon ground turmeric
½ teaspoon garam masala
¼ teaspoon ground cumin

Juice of ½ small lemon
1 tablespoon tomato paste
8 small new potatoes

1. Preheat oven to 350 F.
2. Combine everything except potatoes in a bowl. Mix to a paste.
3. Peel potatoes. Pierce in several places with a skewer or fork. Cut a lengthwise wedge (½ inch wide) out of each potato. Rub the hole with the spice paste, and insert the wedge back in. Rub the potato all over with the remaining paste.
4. Place a rack on a baking tray and arrange the potatoes on the rack. Bake for 30 to 40 minutes, turning every 10 minutes, until tender. Serve at once.

SOUPS

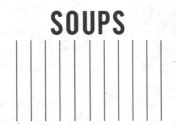

A steam-wreathed tureen of soup, emitting delectable and tantalizing whiffs of comfort, never fails to delight even the grumpiest diner. Soup nourishes the soul as well as the body. It evokes memories of cozy evenings by the hearth, while the cruel winter elements rage outside. Soup slides down soothingly—smooth and easy—making the diner feel loved and indulged. I am happy to tell you that Slim Cuisine soups allow you to wallow in that lovely feeling without wallowing in fat as well. Several Slim Cuisine techniques make this splendid state of affairs possible; use them to reduce the fat and Calorie levels of any soup recipe you might come across:

1. Never use oil, butter, or margarine to sauté the vegetables that form the flavor base of a soup. Use the stock-sauté method, or the onion infusion.

2. The classic way of enriching many soups is with butter, egg yolk, and cream. Don't do it! The best way to enrich a creamy vegetable purée soup is with the vegetable itself. Use more of the vegetable than called for in a traditional recipe. When cooked, purée the soup in a blender or processor, or put it through a food mill. It will be rich and creamy. In some cases, you might want to purée half of the soup, then combine the puréed and unpuréed portions. This makes a lovely, interesting texture.

3. Substitute low-fat fromage blanc, yogurt, quark, or skim milk for sour cream, crème fraîche, or cream.

4. Use potato for body and thickening. It adds plenty of nutrients but few Calories and no fat.

5. Baked vegetables, especially baked garlic, give wonderful depth to low-fat soups. One of the soups in this section is made up entirely of baked vegetables. It is satisfying enough to be a main dish, yet it has only 98 Calories per 1-cup serving! Experiment with adding various puréed baked vegetables to soup for flavor and body.

6. Splash wine and spirits into your soups. In the brisk simmering much of the alcohol (and alcohol Calories) evaporate but the flavor remains. For instance, red wine and cognac combine to add richness to French Onion Soup (page 77). Without them, this extremely low-fat soup would have a somewhat anemic taste.

If you love to begin a meal with a nice hearty bowlful of steaming soup, you will be pleased to know that soup has been shown to be a splendid diet food. Recent research studies at several American universities have suggested that soup, eaten in large quantities before a meal, results in fewer total Calories ingested in that meal. In fact, the more soup, the fewer total Calories. Furthermore, the study suggests that enthusiastic soup eaters who eat the hot, soothing stuff regularly are much more likely to keep to their target weight over the long term than nonsoup eaters.

The blender is used to purée many soups. Never fill the blender jar with hot soup. When the machine is switched on, the hot liquid will surge up, blow off the cover, splash and burn the cook, and make a spectacular mess on the ceiling. Let the soup cool somewhat first, then fill the jar less than halfway.

RED CABBAGE SOUP

 Makes 2 quarts

A dazzlingly purple soup with a homey taste. Perfect cold-weather fare.

½ cup chopped shallots
7½ cups chicken stock
1 medium baking potato, peeled and coarsely chopped
1 medium red cabbage (2 to 2½ pounds), cored and shredded
1 large tart apple, peeled, cored, and coarsely chopped

Salt and freshly ground pepper to taste
4 to 6 tablespoons low-fat yogurt at room temperature
Freshly ground nutmeg

1. Combine shallots and ½ cup stock in a nonreactive soup pot. Cover and bring to a boil.

2. Uncover. Reduce heat slightly and simmer briskly until the liquid has evaporated and the shallots are beginning to stick to the pan.

3. Toss in the potato and an additional splash of stock. Toss, stirring and scraping up the browned bits on the bottom of the pot.

4. When the potato begins to brown slightly, toss in the cabbage and apple. Toss and cook over medium heat for 2 to 3 minutes.

5. Pour in the remaining stock. Season to taste. Bring to a boil, reduce heat, and simmer, partially covered, for 15 minutes, until the cabbage and potatoes are tender but not mushy. Taste and adjust seasoning, and cool slightly.

6. In a blender, purée the soup. Do this in several batches. (The soup may be made in advance to this point and refrigerated for 1 or 2 days.)

7. At serving time, heat the soup until it is piping hot. Serve it in clear glass bowls to show off its gorgeous purple color. Swirl 1 tablespoon of yogurt decoratively over the surface of each serving, and sprinkle on some freshly grated nutmeg.

TURNIP SOUP

♡ ☆ ◔   *Makes 7 cups*

The garlic may seem excessive, but (if the garlic is fresh) there is no vulgar garlicky taste in this soup, just a gentle, nutty sweetness. Although there is no cream, only a few ounces of skim milk, the texture is velvety and creamy. Try this even if you think you hate turnips. The humble root reaches exquisite heights in this soup. The recipe also works well with parsnips, rutabagas, or a combination of root vegetables.

8 cups peeled, coarsely diced small white turnips (about 2½ pounds)
15 large cloves garlic, peeled
5 cups stock

1 orange
½ cup skim milk
Salt and freshly ground pepper to taste

1. Combine the turnips, garlic, and stock in a nonreactive soup pot. Bring to a boil. Skim off the scum.

2. Reduce heat and simmer partially covered until the turnips and garlic are tender, 15 to 20 minutes. Cool slightly.

3. Purée the soup in a blender and return to the pot. The texture should be very smooth and velvety.

4. With a citrus zester, zest the orange rind right over the pot, so that the rind goes in and the orange oil as well. Save the orange flesh for another use (a private nibble, perhaps). Stir in the milk and season to taste. Reheat gently, stirring occasionally. Serve piping hot. (This soup may be made in advance and refrigerated for several days or frozen.)

Variation:

Omit the orange rind. Prepare red pepper purée from Baked or Grilled Red Peppers (page 27). Swirl a blob of red pepper purée decoratively onto the surface of each serving of soup.

BEAN SOUP

Makes 8¾ cups

This is a magnificent and sophisticated soup, full of intriguing textures and tastes in perfect harmony. It has echoes of the culinary traditions of both Mexico and Thailand. Jalapeños are fiery Mexican peppers. Look for small cans of jalapeños in vinegar in specialty shops and some supermarkets. They are to be found where other Mexican foods (chili, tortilla chips, et cetera) are found. The use of canned beans makes the preparation of this soup quick and easy. Always rinse canned beans before using, so that a good proportion of their added salt is washed away.

One 1-pound-12-ounce can Italian tomatoes
One 4-ounce can sliced jalapeños in vinegar, liquid reserved
4½ cups stock
Three 1-pound cans pinto beans, drained and rinsed
1 rounded tablespoon tomato paste
½ teaspoon dried oregano, crumbled, or more to taste
A few grinds of black pepper
½ cup coarsely chopped fresh parsley

Several sprigs fresh coriander, coarsely chopped
1 bunch scallions, trimmed and thinly sliced
1 large clove garlic, minced
4 tablespoons red wine vinegar
6 tablespoons water
Juice of 1 lime, or more to taste
6 tablespoons grated Parmesan cheese, or more to taste
Salt (optional)

1. Pour the tomatoes and their juices into a blender. Add approximately one-quarter of the jalapeños and one-quarter of the jalapeño juice (use less if you want a tame soup, more if you pride yourself on your asbestos palate). Save the remainder of the peppers for another use. Purée. Put the purée through a nonreactive sieve so that the seeds are left behind.

2. Pour the sieved mixture into a nonreactive soup pot. Add the stock, beans, tomato paste, oregano, and pepper. Simmer, uncovered, for 20 minutes. Roughly mash some of the beans in the pot with a potato masher. (The recipe may be made in advance to this point. Cool and refrigerate until needed.)

3. Meanwhile, combine chopped parsley, chopped coriander, scallions, garlic, vinegar, and water in a small saucepan or frying pan. Boil, stirring occasionally, until almost dry. Stir this mixture into the simmering bean soup.

4. Stir in the lime juice. Sprinkle on the Parmesan cheese. Stir gently until the cheese melts into the soup. Taste and add more lime juice, pepper, or oregano to taste. If you feel it needs it, add a bit of salt, but it probably won't need much.

CARROT SOUP

♡ ☆ ◔ ❄   *Makes 8¾ cups*

This burnt-orange soup has two versions: the first elegant, smooth, and piquant; the second chunky, homey, and mild.

1½ pounds carrots, peeled and
  coarsely chopped
2 stalks celery, coarsely chopped
5 cloves garlic, peeled
1 large onion, coarsely chopped
7 cups plus 3 fluid ounces stock
¼ cup dry sherry
1 baking potato, peeled and
  coarsely diced

½ teaspoon ground nutmeg
Freshly ground pepper
Salt to taste
3 tablespoons nonfat yogurt or
  fromage blanc, at room
  temperature
1 rounded tablespoon Dijon
  mustard
1 tablespoon snipped fresh dill

1. Combine carrots, celery, garlic, onion, 3 fluid ounces of stock and half the sherry in a nonreactive soup pot. Cover and bring to a boil. Allow to boil, uncovering to stir occasionally, until almost dry.

2. Uncover. Let cook for a few moments more until the mixture begins to burn just a bit and to stick to the bottom of the pot. Splash in the remaining sherry and boil, scraping up the brown bits on the bottom of the pan with a wooden spoon.

3. Toss in the potato. Cook over medium heat for 1 or 2 minutes, stirring. Stir in the nutmeg and pepper and toss to coat the vegetables with the spices.

4. Stir in 7 cups stock and salt to taste. Cover and bring to a boil. Reduce heat and simmer, partially covered, until the vegetables are tender, 20 to 30 minutes. Cool slightly.

5. Put the soup into the blender in batches. Purée to a smooth, velvety consistency. (The soup may be made in advance to this point. Cool and refrigerate until needed.) Return to the soup pot and bring to a simmer.

6. Remove the soup from the heat. Whisk together the yogurt or fromage blanc and the mustard. Gradually stir some of the soup into the mustard mixture. Then, slowly, stir the mustard-soup mixture back into the soup, along with the dill.

Variation:

Instead of puréeing the soup to a velvety smoothness, pulse the blender on and off a few times, so that the soup is chunky. Omit the fromage blanc and the mustard. Stir in the dill.

RED PEPPER SOUP

 Makes 7 cups

Red peppers are fleshy, sweet, and brilliantly colored. They give all three properties to this gentle soup. Potatoes add additional substance and fromage blanc gives a touch of creaminess with no added fat.

2 medium onions, chopped	8 large red peppers, trimmed,
6 cups stock	ribbed, and coarsely diced
¼ cup dry white wine	1 teaspoon dried thyme,
1 medium baking potato, peeled	crumbled
and coarsely diced	Cayenne pepper to taste
Salt and freshly ground pepper to	Nonfat fromage blanc or yogurt
taste	

1. Combine the onions and ½ cup stock in a soup pot. Cover and bring to a boil. Reduce heat and allow to steam for 5 minutes.

2. Uncover and continue cooking for another few minutes, until the mixture begins to brown and stick to the bottom of the pan. Splash in the wine and boil, scraping the browned bits off the bottom of the pot.

3. Stir in the potato and another ½ cup stock. Cover and cook over medium heat for 5 minutes. While cooking, uncover and stir once or twice. After 5 minutes, splash in a bit more stock and again scrape any browned bits from the bottom of the pot. Season the mixture with a bit of salt and a generous grinding of pepper.

4. Toss in the red peppers, thyme, and a bit of cayenne. Pour in the remaining stock and simmer, partially covered, until the vegetables are tender, about 30 minutes. Let cool.

5. In batches, purée the soup in a blender. Pour it through a fine sieve into the soup pot. Rub the solids through with a wooden spoon or a rubber spatula. The tough pepper skins will be left behind in the sieve. Discard them. (The soup may be cooled at this point, and then refrigerated for a few days or frozen.)

6. Gently heat the soup. Add more salt, black pepper, and cayenne pepper to taste. Crumble in a touch more dried thyme, if desired.

7. Serve with a dollop of yogurt or fromage blanc on each serving.

Variation:

ROASTED PEPPER SOUP

Grill or roast the peppers (page 27). Dice them and add them to the onions in step 1. Simmer briefly. Purée the soup, but there is no need to sieve it. A little roasted garlic purée certainly wouldn't hurt. This soup—as you can imagine—has character.

ONION SOUP

Makes 5 cups

69 Calories per 1¼-cup serving
0.2g fat
(Traditional onion soup: 263 Calories,
13g fat)

French onion soup without butter or oil? Yes, if you utilize two Slim Cuisine techniques: browned onions and scallion/shallot infusion. A good portion of the long cooking time is untended simmering, so you need not feel tied to the stove for the whole time.

8 cups thinly sliced Spanish onions (about 6 large)
5 leeks, cleaned, trimmed, and thinly sliced
2 cups stock
1¼ cups dry red wine
1 tablespoon all-purpose white flour
8 cups stock, brought to a boil
1 piece Parmesan rind
½ cup Cognac
1 bunch trimmed scallions, thinly sliced
3 shallots, chopped
Salt and pepper to taste

1. Combine onions, leeks, and 2 cups stock in a deep soup pot. Cover and bring to a boil. Reduce heat a bit and simmer briskly for 10 minutes.

2. Uncover. Simmer 35 to 40 minutes, stirring occasionally. At this point, the onions will be turning amber-brown and dry. Stir constantly as they cook a few minutes more. They will soon begin to stick and burn. Keep stirring over low heat for about 10 minutes more. As you stir, scrape up the browned bits on the bottom of the pot. Turn up the heat a bit. Splash in one-third of the red wine. Boil until dry, stirring and scraping like mad.

3. Reduce the heat to low and stir in the flour. Stir for about 3 minutes over low heat.

4. Gradually add the hot stock and half the remaining red wine, stirring all the while. Add the Parmesan rind. Partially cover the pot and simmer 40 minutes, skimming and stirring occasionally.

5. During the last 20 minutes, stir in the Cognac. Then combine the scallions, shallots, and the rest of the red wine in a small saucepan or frying pan; bring to a boil, reduce heat, and simmer briskly until almost all liquid has evaporated. Stir this mixture into the simmering soup.

6. When the soup has simmered for 40 minutes, remove from the heat. Season to taste. Remove the Parmesan rind. Serve piping hot.

SOUP OF BAKED VEGETABLES

                            Makes 6 cups

Do not be daunted by the number of steps in this recipe; it is very easy and makes one of the richest most deliciously satisfying soups you have ever eaten. Serve it with crusty bread spread with low-fat quark and you have a meal.

4 small eggplants (about ½ pound each)	Salt and freshly ground pepper to taste
1 large Spanish onion	½ teaspoon dried thyme, crumbled
2 heads garlic	½ teaspoon dried tarragon, crumbled
2 red peppers	¼ teaspoon allspice
One 1-pound-12-ounce can Italian tomatoes, well drained	¼ cup Cognac
1 tablespoon tomato paste	
4 cups stock	

1. Preheat the oven to 425 F. Prick the eggplants in several places with a skewer or the prongs of a fork.

2. Spread the eggplants, onion, garlic, and red peppers on a large baking sheet. Bake for 1 hour. Turn the peppers once or twice during this time.

3. After 1 hour, remove all vegetables except the onion from the oven and allow to cool. The peppers should be quite black. Place them in a paper bag for a few minutes. (If they are not charred all over, place them under the broiler first, turning frequently, until they are thoroughly blackened. Then, remove from broiler and close up in a paper bag.)

4. Place the drained tomatoes in the blender. Cut the stems from the eggplants and strip off the skins. Place the pulp in the blender. Purée. Push the purée through a fine sieve into a soup pot, so that all the tomato and eggplant seeds are left behind. Discard the seeds.

5. Squeeze the garlic cloves so that the softened garlic purée pops from the skins. Add the purée to the pot.

6. Remove the peppers from the bag and strip off the charred skins. Discard the skins and the seeds. Purée the peppers in the blender, and add them to the pot.

7. By this time, the onion will be soft. Remove it from the oven. (Work with a mitt; the onion will be hot!) Cut off the stem and root ends from the onion and strip off the first 2 layers. Cut it into quarters and place in the blender and purée. Add this to the pot.

8. Stir in the tomato paste, stock, and all the herbs and seasonings. Simmer, partially covered, for 30 minutes, stirring occasionally.

9. Stir in the Cognac and simmer for 5 minutes more. Serve piping hot. This soup may be prepared 2 days ahead and refrigerated or frozen. The flavor will improve each day.

🕒 ▭ Prepare eggplants, garlic, and onion in the microwave. Use jarred peppers.

SPLIT PEA SOUP

❄

Makes 6¼ cups

The baked garlic is optional in this hearty soup, but I strongly recommend that you try it; it gives a wonderful dimension to the pale green brew. The soup can be made in advance, but it will thicken dramatically in the refrigerator. Thin it with stock before reheating. This soup works particularly well with a stock made from the carcass of a smoked chicken or turkey.

½ pound split peas, rinsed and
   picked over
2 baking potatoes, peeled and
   cubed
8 cups stock
1 large onion, chopped

Purée from 1 or 2 heads Baked
   Garlic (page 23) (optional)
4 tablespoons grated Parmesan
   cheese
Salt to taste

1. Combine peas, potatoes, and 4 cups stock in a saucepan. Bring
to boil, reduce heat, and simmer briskly, partially covered, until peas
and potatoes are tender, about 40 minutes. Cool slightly.

2. While the vegetables are simmering, sauté the onion in stock
according to the Slim Cuisine method: combine onions and ½ cup
stock in a frying pan. Cover and bring to a boil. Uncover and boil for
5 minutes or so, until the liquid has almost cooked away. Reduce heat
and simmer until the onions are just about dry and beginning to stick
and burn. Pour in a splash of stock and boil, stirring and scraping up
the browned bits on the bottom of the frying pan.

3. When the peas and potatoes are tender, push them through a
fine sieve or put them through a food mill and return them to the pot.
Add the sautéed onions and the remaining stock and stir in the garlic
purée, if used.

4. Simmer the soup for approximately 15 minutes. Add the cheese
and stir gently until it melts into the soup. Taste and add a touch of
salt, if needed. Serve piping hot.

WILD MUSHROOM SOUP

                    Makes 5 cups

The dried mushrooms are available in gourmet shops and specialty
food shops. Chinese and Japanese dried mushrooms may be substituted if necessary. The soup may be made a few days in advance. If
fresh oyster mushrooms are available, use them as part of the measure
of fresh mushrooms. They will impart a lovely, buttery quality to the
soup. And if fresh shiitakes are available, use a few of those as well.

1 ounce dried cèpes *(Boletus edulis)*
½ ounce dried morels
2 pounds fresh mushrooms, cleaned and quartered
About 1¼ cups medium sherry
1 or 2 dashes low-sodium soy sauce

½ cup chopped shallots
2 cloves garlic, minced
1 teaspoon dried tarragon, crumbled
7 to 8 cups stock
Salt and pepper to taste
Piece of Parmesan cheese rind

1. Rinse dried mushrooms well under cold running water. Put them in a bowl with hot water to cover generously. Let soak for 1 hour.

2. In a heavy large nonstick frying pan, combine the fresh mushrooms with the sherry and soy sauce. If your frying pan is too small, do this step in several batches. Simmer briskly until the mixture is almost dry. Stir frequently and do not let the mushrooms scorch or brown. Scrape the mixture into a large pot.

3. Strain the soaking water from the dried mushrooms through a sieve lined with cheesecloth or a coffee filter to eliminate grit and sand. Rinse the mushrooms well under cold running water. Discard any tough stems and chop the mushrooms coarsely.

4. Add the soaked mushrooms and their filtered water to the fresh mushrooms in the pot.

5. In a small frying pan, combine the shallots, garlic, tarragon, ½ cup stock, and a splash of sherry. Boil until almost dry. Add mixture to the pot.

6. Add the remaining stock, a bit of salt and pepper, and the Parmesan rind. Bring to a boil, reduce heat, and simmer, partially covered, for 1 hour. Discard the cheese rind. Taste and add more salt and pepper, if necessary. Cool. In batches, put the soup in the blender. Flick the motor on and off once or twice (you want a rough-chopped effect, *not* a smooth purée). Serve piping hot. The soup will keep in the refrigerator for several days and may be frozen.

CHESTNUT SOUP

Makes 7 cups

This is a soup for special occasions, a rich starter for a gala meal. The use of canned chestnuts (available in gourmet shops and many supermarkets) makes it very easy to prepare. Happily, chestnuts, unlike other nuts, are very low in fat.

6 shallots, chopped
¾ pound carrots, peeled and
  chopped
1 large celery stalk, chopped
7½ cups stock
1 cup dry red wine

4 cups canned unsweetened
  chestnuts, drained
Salt and freshly ground pepper to
  taste
¼ teaspoon freshly grated nutmeg
1 cup skim milk

1. Combine the shallots, carrots, celery, ½ cup stock, and ½ cup wine in a soup pot. Cover, bring to a boil, and continue to boil until almost all the liquid is cooked away.

2. Add the chestnuts, remaining stock, and seasonings. Simmer, covered, for 45 minutes to 1 hour, until the chestnuts and vegetables are very tender. Cool slightly.

3. Purée the soup in a blender, then return it to the soup pot and stir in the milk. Return to a simmer and simmer for 10 minutes. The soup may be served at once, or cooled and refrigerated for serving up to 3 days later.

4. To serve, bring to a simmer, stir in the remaining ½ cup wine, and simmer for a few minutes.

ITALIAN SAUSAGE SOUP

Makes 12 cups

This one-pot meal is more of a stew than a soup. It provides lavish comfort on a cold, wintry evening. Eat it in front of the fire. Serve a crusty rustic whole-grain loaf with it. The soup reheats very well—in fact, it improves in flavor if made a day or so ahead.

2 large onions, coarsely chopped
3 cloves garlic, crushed
6¼ cups stock
One 1-pound-12-ounce can plum tomatoes, drained and crushed with the hands
1½ cups dry red wine
1 teaspoon dried basil, crumbled
1 teaspoon dried oregano, crumbled
1 piece Parmesan cheese rind
1 small red pepper, peeled, seeded, ribbed, and coarsely diced

3 small zucchini, trimmed and sliced ½ inch thick
½ cup tiny pasta shells
Salt and freshly ground pepper to taste
4 tablespoons chopped fresh parsley
25 cooked Italian Sausage Balls (page 105)
One 15-ounce can cannellini beans, rinsed and drained
Grated Parmesan cheese

1. Sauté onions and garlic in ¾ cup stock according to the Slim Cuisine technique (see page 15) until amber-brown and tender. Stir in tomatoes, wine, remaining stock, herbs, and Parmesan rind. Simmer briskly, uncovered, for 15 minutes.

2. Add the red pepper, zucchini, pasta, salt, and pepper. Cover. Simmer for 10 minutes, or until the pasta and vegetables are tender. Stir occasionally.

3. Add the chopped parsley, sausage balls, and beans. Heat through. Discard the Parmesan rind. Serve piping hot. Pass around grated Parmesan cheese at the table.

CHILLED CORN SOUP

Makes 5 cups

This recipe is adapted from the Roux brothers, my gastronomic heroes. I specify a frying pan—an odd utensil for soup—but you will find that the skim milk is less likely to scorch and overflow in a frying pan than in a saucepan.

1 small onion, halved and sliced into thin half-moons	Pinch nutmeg
½ cup stock	Salt to taste
12 ounces corn kernels	Pinch paprika
3½ cups skim milk	Snipped chives

1. In a frying pan sauté the onion in the stock according to the Slim Cuisine technique (see page 15).
2. If the corn kernels are canned, rinse and drain them. Add them to the onion and stir. Pour in the milk, season with nutmeg and a bit of salt. Gently and slowly bring mixture to a boil. Simmer for 5 minutes. Cool slightly.
3. Purée the mixture in the blender, then rub it through a sieve. Chill.
4. Serve with a sprinkling of paprika and snipped chives on each serving.

Variation:

MEXICAN CORN SOUP

Add ground cumin, cayenne pepper, and a pinch of crumbled dried oregano in step 2. Omit the nutmeg. In step 4 omit the paprika and chives. Garnish instead with chopped fresh coriander and a sprinkling of chili powder.

JELLIED GAZPACHO

Serves 10

This trembling red jelly, studded with jewellike bits of vegetables and herbs, is fragrant, vivid, and exciting. Serve it spooned into clear glass bowls. It can be eaten with a spoon or spread onto crackers.

1 small can plus 1 large can Italian plum tomatoes with juice (2 pounds 10 ounces total)
4 teaspoons unflavored gelatin
6 ounces tomato paste
Juice of ½ lemon
¼ cup white wine vinegar
Salt and pepper to taste
Dash cayenne pepper (optional)
1 teaspoon chopped fresh oregano

1 teaspoon chopped fresh basil
1 clove garlic, crushed
½ cup thinly sliced scallions
½ yellow pepper, minced
¼ cucumber, peeled, seeded, and minced
½ cup chopped fresh parsley
2 canned plum tomatoes, seeded, well drained, and chopped (in summer, use fresh tomatoes)

1. Blend the tomatoes, juice and all, in a blender, then sieve them. You should end up with 3¾ cups of tomato juice. Save any extra for another use. Measure out ¾ cup and put it in a nonreactive saucepan. Bring just to a simmer. Immediately remove from the heat.

2. Sprinkle the gelatin into the hot tomato juice. Stir well to dissolve. Add the remaining tomato juice, tomato paste, lemon juice, vinegar, salt, pepper, and cayenne, if used. Stir very well. Let stand for an hour or so, until the mixture is beginning to thicken.

3. Fold in the remaining ingredients. Pour the mixture into a large bowl. Cover and chill thoroughly.

FISH

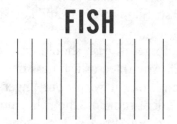

This section deals very specifically with techniques. There are countless ways of seasoning, saucing, and serving fish. Once you learn the Slim Cuisine techniques of fish cooking, let your imagination run wild.

A fish dinner is my idea of culinary heaven. The delicacy of fish and its ability to "marry" with a large spectrum of flavorful ingredients make finned creatures my first choice of main course for special dinner parties and celebration meals. A word of warning, however: When fish is overcooked or kept several days past its prime, it is fit for no one but a not very fastidious cat. Fish should be sparklingly fresh and *just* cooked so that it is moist, succulent, and sweetly flavorful.

Secrets of Perfect Fish Cookery

To cook fish properly, cook it quickly. Do not "cook until it flakes easily," as many recipes direct. Instead, cook it until it turns opaque and just barely begins to flake. It should retain the faint sweet taste and moisture of the sea or stream. To achieve the proper effect, follow this foolproof rule of thumb developed by the Canadian Fisheries Board: With a ruler, measure the fish at its thickest point. Cook the fish (under a broiler, in the oven, or in a frying pan) at high heat for 10 minutes per inch of thickness. Thus, if the fish is ½ inch thick or less it will cook for 5 minutes, 1½ inches for 15 minutes, and so on.

To Buy Fresh Fish

All the careful timing and exquisite seasoning in the world are useless when applied to old fish. Shop carefully and keep these points in mind:

1. If it smells fishy, forget it! Fish should have a faint, clean odor of the sea or the stream. Any trace of fishiness means old fish.
2. Fresh fish is firm. Poke it with your finger. If the flesh springs back it is fresh. If the dent remains, the fish is not for you.
3. A fish fillet should not shred or tear when held up. And fillets should never feel slimy.
4. Fish that has been stored improperly or too long develops sunken, milky, filmed eyes. Choose fish with bulging, bright, staring eyes, however unnerving that stare may be.
5. If the proprietor of the fish market does not allow you to poke, prod, and smell the wares, consider finding another market.

Fish Facts

Fish makes a perfect main dish from a nutritional standpoint, as well as a gastronomic one. Low in calories and sodium, high in protein and B vitamins, it is a dietitian's dream. The fat content of fish varies with the species, but even fattier fish is relatively low in calories, and fish fat is entirely different from animal fat. Recent scientific and medical studies in several different countries suggest that fish oils seem to have a protective effect on the heart. Frequent fish meals, coupled with an otherwise low-fat diet, may well help reduce the risk of heart disease.

Slim Cuisine Methods of Cooking Fish

Use no fats and oils and (it should go without saying) abandon all thoughts of deep-frying. For the sake of good taste, avoid blanketing fish in thick tomato sauces, or excessive showerings of dried herbs. Keep it simple so that the fresh, vibrant taste of the fish itself shines through.

TO STEAM FISH IN PARCHMENT

♡ ⏲

Steaming fish *en papillote* (in paper packets) is a classic method that lends itself perfectly to Slim Cuisine. The fish steams in its own juices and emerges spectacularly succulent and luscious. Keep the seasoning fresh and simple. For each piece of fish use a tablespoon of dry white wine, sherry, or white vermouth, a tablespoon of lemon juice and a scattering of chopped fresh herbs. Try parsley, scallions, and minced fresh ginger; basil or mint and minced garlic; thyme, tarragon, and slivered orange zest; coriander, lime juice, and slivered lime zest; ginger, scallions, and low-sodium soy sauce. Chopped or sliced mushrooms can be added, too. Find combinations that please you and those you feed.

1. Use fish steaks, fillets, or small whole fish, such as trout, gutted and boned. (When using whole fish, remove the head and tail, if desired. Some flavor will be lost with the head but you will be spared the baleful stare.) Rinse the fish and dry it on paper towels. With tweezers or a small pair of pliers, pull out any small bones that remain in the fillets or boneless whole fish.

2. With a ruler, measure the fish at its thickest point. (Be sure to measure its *depth*, not its length!) Jot down the inches of thickness.

3. For each piece of fish, tear a piece of parchment paper large enough to enclose the piece generously. Place each portion of fish on a piece of paper (fillets should be skin side down) near the bottom edge. Season with appropriate herbs, spices, citrus juice, and spirits (see suggestions above). Fold the paper over the fish. The outer edges of the paper should be even. Crimp the paper closed over the fish as follows: fold down one corner; start a second fold so that it incorporates a bit of the first fold; continue folding and crimping all around until the fish is well secured and no steam or juice can escape. Make sure you leave space on top so that the paper does not touch the top surface of the fish.

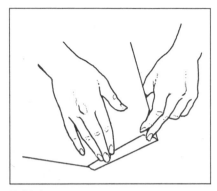

Fold down one corner.

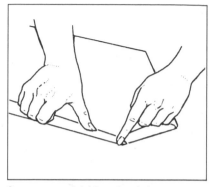

Start a second fold so that it incorporates a bit of the first fold.

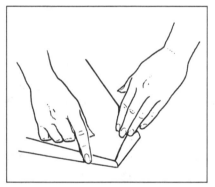

Continue folding and crimping all around until

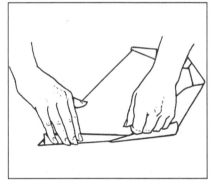

the fish is well secured and no steam or juice can escape.

Make sure you leave space on top so that the paper does not touch the top surface of the fish.

4. Preheat the oven to 450 F. Place the fish packets, in one layer, on a baking sheet. Bake for 10 minutes per inch of thickness. The packets will become browned and puffy.

5. Give each diner a packet and a pair of scissors. When the packets are cut, the perfumed steam will imbue the air, delighting all present.

To Broil Fish

Years ago when I was visiting friends in Maine, I learned to coat fish fillets with a thin layer of mayonnaise before broiling, to keep them beautifully moist. It works with Slim Cuisine "Mayonnaise," too. For fish, I make the mayonnaise with a mixture of 2 parts yogurt to 1 part Dijon mustard. In the broiling, the coating turns fluffy and the fish stays moist and pearly.

BROILED SOLE WITH MUSTARD

Serves 4

White wine	2 tablespoons low-fat yogurt
4 fillets sole or flounder	Freshly ground pepper to taste
1 tablespoon Dijon mustard	

1. Preheat the broiler to its highest setting.
2. Pour the wine into the broiler pan to a depth of ⅙ inch
3. Place the fillets in one layer in the pan. (They should not touch each other.)
4. Combine the mustard, yogurt, and pepper. Spread mixture evenly over each fillet.
5. Broil 4 to 5 inches from the heat for 5 minutes. Serve at once.

OVEN-POACHED FISH

1. Preheat the oven to 450 F.
2. With a ruler, measure the fish at its thickest point (be sure to measure its *depth*, not its length!). Jot down the inches of thickness.

3. Pour dry white wine or dry vermouth into a shallow baking dish to a depth of ⅛₆ inch. Place the fish steaks or fish fillets (skin side down) in the wine in one layer (they should not touch each other). Season to taste or as indicated in the individual recipe. The seasoning suggestions for fish *en papillote* (94) also apply to steamed fish and to poached fish. Cover each piece of fish with a lettuce leaf. (This keeps the fish from drying out.) Bake for 10 minutes per inch of thickness. Discard the lettuce leaves, and serve at once.

OVEN-"FRIED" FISH

♡ ⏲

126 Calories per 3½ ounces (of cod)
0.6g fat
(Traditional fried cod: 200 Calories per
3½ ounces, 10.3g fat)

1. Preheat oven to 500 F.

2. Choose haddock or cod fillets. With a ruler, measure the fillet at its thickest point. (Be sure to measure its *depth*, not its length!) Jot down the inches of thickness.

3. Dip one side of the fillets (not the skin side) into buttermilk or yogurt, then dredge them in seasoned bread crumbs. (Make your own: The packaged kind tend to be awful. Season them with salt and pepper and any herbs and spices you like.) The fish should be very well coated.

4. Place a rack on a flat baking sheet. Put the fillets, breaded side up, on the rack in one layer (they should not touch each other). Bake for 10 minutes per inch of thickness. Serve at once with lemon wedges. This fish is particularly good on a bed of Helen's Terracotta Sauce (page 162).

STEAMED FISH FILLETS

Serves 4

Lettuce leaves
4 fish fillets (about 6 ounces each)
   white fish or salmon
2 tablespoons dry white wine or
   vermouth, or 2 tablespoons
   fresh lemon or lime juice
3 tablespoons finely minced
   shallots or thinly sliced
   scallions

2 tablespoons chopped fresh
   parsley
1 tablespoon chopped fresh herbs,
   such as tarragon, thyme,
   marjoram, or chervil
Salt and freshly ground pepper

1. Line a steamer rack with lettuce leaves. Arrange the fish fillets, skin side down, in one layer on the leaves. Sprinkle them evenly with all the remaining ingredients. Have water boiling in the bottom of the steamer.

2. Put the rack in the steamer, cover, and steam the fish over boiling water for 10 minutes per inch of thickness. Serve at once.

Suggestions for Steamed, Poached, or "Fried" Fish

Serve the fish fillets on a bed of: Rémoulade Sauce (page 66); Tzatziki (page 63); Red or Yellow Pepper Sauce (page 133), or coat the plate with half yellow pepper sauce, half red, before positioning the fish; Creamy Dill Pesto (page 160); or Helen's Terracotta Sauce (page 162).

SOLE EN PAPILLOTE

♡ ◔   *Serves 4*

1 large Spanish onion, halved and
   sliced into paper-thin half-
   moons
½ cup stock
4 fillets sole
Salt and freshly ground pepper to
   taste

2 tablespoons chopped fresh
   tarragon, or 1 teaspoon dried
2 tablespoons chopped chives or
   thinly sliced scallions

1. Preheat oven to 450 F.

2. Sauté the onion in stock according to the Slim Cuisine method (see page 15), until amber-brown and meltingly tender.

3. Place each fillet on a square of parchment paper large enough to enclose it. Season each fillet with salt and pepper, and top with an equal amount of herbs. Put some of the sautéed onions on top of each fillet.

4. Seal the packets and cook according to the master recipe (page 89). Serve at once.

COD EN PAPILLOTE

♡ ◔   *Serves 4*

Here is a lovely, fresh, simple way to cook cod in parchment-paper packets; just one example of how this method can produce a quick but extremely elegant main dish. Serve it with steamed new potatoes and a green salad tossed with one of the Slim Cuisine dressings (see pages 202–203).

4 cod fillets (4 ounces each) (choose fillets that are of equal thickness)
4 generous tablespoons chopped fresh parsley
4 generous tablespoons chopped fresh mint

4 tablespoons fresh lemon juice
4 tablespoons dry white vermouth
Salt and freshly ground pepper to taste

1. Preheat the oven to 450 F.

2. Measure the thickness of the cod fillets. Place each fillet on a sheet of parchment paper.

3. Sprinkle 1 tablespoon each of parsley, mint, lemon juice, vermouth, and some salt and pepper over each fillet. Enclose the fillets in the paper according to the directions in the master recipe (page 89).

4. Place the packets on a baking sheet and bake for 10 minutes per inch of thickness. Serve at once, right from the packets.

MEAT

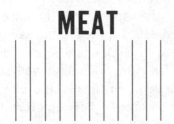

There is no need to cut out red meat, in fact it is wise not to. Meat is an excellent source of nutrition: high-quality protein, B vitamins, zinc and other important trace minerals, iron, and more. In fact, the iron from meat is absorbed more readily into the body than the iron in any other foodstuff or iron supplement. Of course, meat is also a source of fat, much of it (although not all of it) saturated. So the trick is to eliminate as much of that fat as possible.

Here are the guidelines:

1. Buy the leanest meat possible. Flank steak—for instance, a paddle-shaped flat steak—is extremely lean and makes a wonderfully satisfying steak dinner. Beef fillet steak is lean, as is pork tenderloin. Always trim away all visible fat before cooking.

2. Rethink the *amount* of meat you eat at one meal. Serve plenty of vegetables and grains with smaller portions of meat. Do as the Chinese do, and make meat more of an accent than a main event. And there is certainly no need to eat meat every day. Eat poultry, fish, dairy, and vegetarian meals as well.

3. Ground meat is a great favorite of mine. Some of the most comforting and delicious dishes in the world—meatballs, meat sauce, shepherd's pie, chili con carne—are made with ground meat. Always buy very lean ground meat, whether it is beef, pork, lamb, or veal. The ideal is to buy a piece of extremely lean meat from the butcher and have him grind it.

4. Never brown ground meat in added fat. Use a nonstick frying pan and let it brown in its own juices. Then drain it very well in a colander over a bowl. (Pour the drained juices into a measuring cup and refrigerate; when they are chilled, the fat will have risen to the surface and congealed. Discard the fat, but save the remaining juices to enrich future stews, casseroles, and sauces.) Even very lean meat will render plenty of fat. After draining it well, spread it out on paper towels, cover with more paper towels, and blot. Blot the frying pan also. Then, when all possible fat has been removed, return the meat to the pan and proceed with the recipe.

5. Stews are disastrous when made from very lean meat. Use beef chuck and trim off surrounding fat. Never brown the meat cubes in fat or oil when beginning a stew. Simply combine the ingredients and braise slowly and gently. During stewing, the meat cubes will release lots of fat. Refrigerate the stew overnight, or quick-chill the juices in the freezer. The fat will rise to the top and harden. Scrape off every speck of fat and discard it.

Meatballs

Tiny, succulent meatballs are delightful. Traditional meatballs are distressingly high in Calories and fat, but it is easy to remedy this. Slim Cuisine techniques result in meatballs that are much more delicate and refined than those made by the bad old methods. In fact, they are more like light and fluffy dumplings than meatballs. Instead of eggs (the yolk is extremely high in fat), puréed baked eggplant is combined with the ground meat. There is no taste, no look, no evidence whatsoever of eggplant in the final cooked meatballs. The vegetable pulp imparts an exquisite lightness, but otherwise there is no sign of that pulp at all.

Instead of frying the meatballs in olive oil, butter, or other highly unsuitable fat, Slim Cuisine calls for quick broiling or sautéing in stock. The choice is yours, and both methods will work beautifully for lamb, beef, or pork. Traditional meatball recipes call for fairly high-fat ground meat. Obviously for these recipes you will use the leanest meat possible.

BROILED LAMB MEATBALLS

❄

Makes 35 nut-size meatballs

18 Calories per meatball
0.3g fat
(Traditional meatballs: 88.2 Calories per
meatball, 5g fat)

These meatballs are good in Tomato Sauce (page 166), a lovely addition to pasta dishes, splendid with Steamed Asparagus (page 177) and Red or Yellow Pepper Sauce (page 133), or try them stuffed into pita bread with Stir-"Fried" Yellow and Red Peppers (page 179) or Cucumber Raita (page 203).

1 pound lean ground lamb
1 small eggplant (¾ to 1 pound),
   baked and puréed or chopped
   fine (see page 28)
3 cloves garlic, minced
½ cup chopped fresh mint (see
   note)
½ cup chopped fresh parsley

1 rounded tablespoon tomato
   paste
Juice and grated rind of 1 small
   lemon
½ cup bread crumbs
Salt and freshly ground pepper to
   taste

1. Place ground lamb in a bowl. Add remaining ingredients. Mix with your hands until thoroughly combined. Fry a tiny test piece (use no fat!) in a small, nonstick frying pan. Taste, then adjust seasonings in the meat mixture to your liking.

2. Preheat the broiler to its highest setting.

3. With your hands, roll the mixture into small balls, each a little smaller than a walnut. You will have approximately 35 in all. Line the broiler pan with foil, shiny side up. Put a rack on the broiler pan, and place the meatballs on the rack.

4. When the broiler is very hot, broil the meatballs 1 inch from the heat for 5 to 7 minutes, until browned on top and just cooked through (no need to turn them). Remove them very gently with tongs and a spatula. Blot the meatballs on paper towels to eliminate any trace of fat, and serve. The meatballs may be made in advance and refriger-

ated or frozen. To reheat, place them in a shallow frying pan with some warm stock. Simmer gently, covered, for 5 to 7 minutes. (Don't boil. The surface of the stock should barely move.) Fish them out very gently with a slotted spoon.

🕐 ⬜ Prepare the eggplant in the microwave (page 28).

Note: For a variation in taste, you can substitute ½ tablespoon fennel seeds, or 1 tablespoon grated fresh ginger, or ½ cup chopped fresh coriander for the mint.

❄ # SAUTÉED VEAL MEATBALLS

Makes 35 meatballs

Elegant, delicate, and exquisite. Sautéing in stock is more difficult and fussy than broiling, but it is worth the effort. Of course, you can broil these if you wish.

1 pound lean ground veal
1 small eggplant (¾ to 1 pound), baked and puréed or chopped fine (see page 28)
Garlic Purée from 1 head of baked garlic (page 25)
1 rounded tablespoon tomato paste
½ cup dry bread crumbs

2 tablespoons chopped fresh parsley
Salt and freshly ground pepper to taste
Juice and grated rind of 1 small lemon
6 tablespoons freshly grated Parmesan cheese
Chicken stock

1. Combine all the ingredients except the chicken stock. Use your hands to mix it all gently but thoroughly. Fry a tiny piece of the mixture in a nonstick frying pan (use no fat!) and taste. Adjust the seasonings to your liking.

2. Form the mixture into balls that are a bit smaller than walnuts.

Heat a large, heavy, nonstick frying pan. Pour in some stock to just film the bottom. Add some of the veal balls. Do not crowd them. You will need to do this in several batches.

3. Let them get crusty, loosening them with a spatula and turning them with tongs, so that they brown on all sides. (Be gentle, they are fragile.) When they are browned and crusty all over, add a bit more stock and simmer for 2 to 3 minutes, turning them, until just cooked through. Blot the balls on paper towels, then spread them in a wide, shallow dish. Repeat until all the meat is used. Add more stock, as needed. When all the veal balls are done, cover well with plastic wrap and refrigerate until needed. (They may be prepared to this point 3 days ahead.)

4. To serve, pour ½ inch of stock into a deep nonstick frying pan. Add the veal balls in one layer. Cover and simmer for 10 minutes or so, until heated through.

🕐 ⬛ Prepare the eggplant in the microwave (page 28).

Note: To broil the veal meatballs, follow the directions for broiling the lamb meatballs (page 99) with this difference: broil for 4 minutes, turn *very* carefully (they are quite fragile), and broil for approximately 4 minutes on the second side.

MEXICAN FRIJOL-ALBONDIGA CASSEROLE

❄️   *Serves 6*

What a festive dish: Mexican baked beans with spicy meatballs. For a lively dinner party, serve this dish with Chilaquiles (page 145), steamed rice, and Stir-"Fried" Zucchini with Lime and Cumin (page 175). Begin with Jellied Gazpacho (page 85) or Chilled Corn Soup (page 84) and end with Mango Sorbet (page 224).

BEANS

Makes 4 cups

1 large onion, chopped
2 large cloves garlic, crushed
½ teaspoon dried oregano,
  crumbled
½ teaspoon chili powder
¾ teaspoon ground cumin
¾ cup stock
1 teaspoon Dijon mustard
One 1-pound can cannellini
  beans, rinsed and drained

One 1-pound can red kidney or
  pinto beans, rinsed and drained
1 canned green chili, chopped
One 1-pound can chopped
  tomatoes
2 tablespoons chopped fresh
  parsley
Salt to taste

1. In a large frying pan, combine the onion, garlic, herbs, spices, and stock. Boil until the mixture is almost dry.

2. Stir in the mustard, beans, chopped chili, tomatoes, parsley, and salt. Simmer gently, stirring occasionally, for 15 to 20 minutes, until thick.

ALBONDIGAS

Makes 38 meatballs

1 pound very lean ground veal or
  pork
Pulp from 1 baked eggplant (¾ to
  1 pound), peeled and chopped
  (see page 28)
2 scallions, chopped
½ cup whole wheat bread crumbs
1 tablespoon chopped fresh mint
  or coriander

½ teaspoon ground cumin
Salt and freshly ground pepper to
  taste
Juice and grated rind of ½ lime
1 tablespoon tomato paste
2 canned green chiles, minced
Several dashes Tabasco sauce

1. Preheat the broiler. Line the broiler tray with foil, shiny side up. Place the broiler rack on the tray.

2. Combine all meatball ingredients in a bowl. Mix well with your hands until well blended. Fry a tiny piece of the mixture in a small nonstick frying pan (use no fat!) and taste. Adjust seasonings to your taste.

3. Form the mixture into tiny balls, a little smaller than walnuts, and arrange them on the broiler rack. Broil close to the heat for 4 minutes on each side. Follow the directions for broiling lamb meatballs (page 99).

TO ASSEMBLE

Stock | 1 tablespoon Parmesan cheese

1. Preheat the oven to 350 F.

2. Spread the beans on the bottom of a shallow baking dish. Add enough stock to make a slightly soupy mixture. Place the albondigas on the bean mixture, pushing them in as you do so. Sprinkle the Parmesan cheese over everything, and cover the dish.

3. Bake for 20 to 30 minutes, until hot and bubbly.

KOFTA CURRY

Makes about 30 meatballs

148 Calories per serving
1.9g fat
(Traditional kofta curry: 591 Calories per
serving, 42.8g fat)

Little meatballs, how I love them! Remember the Slim Cuisine technique of adding chopped baked eggplant to the meat. There will be no eggplant taste, but the Calories in each meatball will be reduced, and the meatballs will be tender and juicy even though the meat is very lean. Of all the curry recipes developed for this book, my tasters loved this one the best. It reheats well from both the refrigerator and the freezer.

MEATBALLS

2 to 3 cloves garlic, minced
Pulp from 1 baked eggplant (see page 28)
1 pound very lean ground lamb or lean ground beef
½ teaspoon ground cinnamon

Pinch ground cloves
½ tablespoon finely grated fresh ginger
Salt to taste
½ cup chopped fresh parsley or coriander

SAUCE

2 large onions, cut into eighths
2 cups stock
2 cloves garlic, minced
½ teaspoon ground turmeric
½ teaspoon ground cinnamon

2 teaspoons ground coriander
Pinch cayenne pepper, or to taste
3 tablespoons tomato paste
Salt to taste

1. Preheat the broiler to its highest setting.

2. In a large bowl, combine the meatball ingredients. Mix with your hands until thoroughly combined. Fry a tiny piece of the mixture in a small frying pan (use no fat!) and taste. Adjust seasonings to your liking. Form the mixture into small balls, a little smaller than walnuts.

3. Line the broiler tray with foil, shiny side up. Place a rack on the tray and arrange the meatballs on it. Broil 1 inch from the heat for 5 minutes, until crusty brown on top. Set aside.

4. Separate the segments of the onion pieces. Spread them in a heavy, nonreactive frying pan. Add *no* liquid or fat. Heat the frying pan gently. Cook at moderate heat, without stirring, for 7 to 10 minutes, until the onions are sizzling and beginning to stick to the pan.

5. Stir in 1¼ cups stock and let it bubble up, stirring up the browned bits with a wooden spoon as it bubbles. Stir in the garlic and spices. Simmer gently, stirring all the while, until the mixture is very thick (not at all soupy). Don't rush this step; it is essential that the spices cook properly. Taste the mixture. The spices should not have a raw, harsh taste. Cook very gently for a few more minutes, if necessary.

6. Stir in the tomato paste and the remaining ¾ cup stock. Place the meatballs in this sauce. Simmer gently, covered, for 15 to 20 minutes, until the sauce is very thick and rich. Salt to taste and serve at once, or cool and refrigerate until needed. This tastes good on the second or third day, so do not hesitate to make it in advance. Add more stock when reheating.

🕐 ▭   Prepare the eggplant in the microwave (page 28).

❄   # ITALIAN SAUSAGE BALLS

Makes 35 sausage balls

25 Calories per sausage ball
0.2g fat
(Traditional Italian sausage:
105 Calories per ounce, 8g fat)

Sausage is a savory mixture of ground pork and pork fat stuffed into animal-intestine casings. The seasonings change with the type of sausage and the region of its origin: nutmeg and mace for German bratwurst; marjoram and garlic for Polish kielbasa; garlic and red pepper for Spanish chorizo; cinnamon, allspice, and orange peel for Greek *loukanika*; sage and thyme for English butcher's sausage.

Use the technique for Slim Cuisine meatballs (page 98) to produce juicy, well-flavored sausage meat without the fat. Pork is bred to be leaner and leaner these days. It should be no problem obtaining a lean piece at the butcher: Have him grind it for you. Or buy lean ground pork from the supermarket. Instead of stuffing the sausage mixture into casings, form it into balls and broil. Even though the meat is lean, it still has some fat in it, which drips off nicely in the broiling. This recipe is for one of my favorites: Italian sausage with crushed dried chiles and fennel seeds. I learned everything I know (or knew) about classic Italian sausage from my old friend, sausage maker Paul Masselli, the Atlanta, Georgia, Picasso of pork butts; and my old teacher, the late Mr. Tammaro, who was a traditional Italian pork butcher in Cambridge, Massachusetts. What *would* they say to this Slim Cuisine variation: *very* lean pork with roasted eggplant pulp replacing the usual pork fat? I hope—after their initial disbelief—they would say "What a fantastic idea; these are *good!*" Substitute any seasonings you like to produce your favorite sausages. And, if you wish, make your sausages with beef or veal, or a combination of meats.

1 pound lean ground pork
2 to 3 small eggplants (about ½ pound each), baked, skinned, and puréed (see page 28)
1 teaspoon fennel or anise seeds
¼ teaspoon crushed dried chiles
3 cloves garlic, crushed to a paste with a mallet

4 tablespoons finely chopped fresh parsley
3 tablespoons dry red wine
Salt and freshly ground pepper to taste

1. Thoroughly mix together all the ingredients, until well combined. Fry a tiny test piece of the mixture (use no fat!) in a small, nonstick frying pan. Taste, then adjust seasonings in the meat mixture to your liking.

2. Preheat the broiler to its highest setting.

3. With your hands, roll the mixture into small balls, each a little smaller than a walnut. Line the broiler pan with foil, shiny side up. Put a rack on the broiler pan, and place the sausage balls on the rack.

4. When the broiler is very hot, broil the sausage balls 1 inch from the heat for 5 minutes. Turn them, and broil for 2 minutes on the second side. Blot the balls on paper towels to remove any trace of fat. Refrigerate until needed. To reheat the sausage balls, use stock as described on page 98.

Sausage Ideas

1. Combine the Italian Sausage Balls with Grilled or Stir-"Fried" Peppers (pages 105 and 27), Sautéed Mushrooms (page 20), and Tomato Sauce (page 160) and serve with pasta or stuffed into crusty rolls. Italian Sausage Balls in Tomato Sauce freeze very well.

2. Serve Sausage Balls with mashed potatoes and Browned Onions (page 16).

3. Serve Sausage Balls with Sautéed Mushrooms (page 20) and broiled tomatoes. What a breakfast!

Ground Meat

I'd rather have ground meat than steak. When I'm hungry for "home cooking," for something warm and satisfying and evocative of happy childhood days, give me ground meat every time. It's amazing the interesting things you can do with it. The following collection of recipes covers the United Kingdom, India, the United States, and Italy.

HAMBURGERS

❄

Makes 4 generous burgers

161 Calories per burger
2.5g fat
(Traditional hamburger: 330 Calories,
23g fat)

Imagine a huge hamburger—juicy and meaty—festooned with shreds of caramelized onions and doused in a thick, spicy red sauce, nesting between the halves of a wheaty bun. Sounds marvelous but quite forbidden, doesn't it? Not to worry. The Slim Cuisine burger is juicy and even more flavorful than the fattening original.

12 ounces finely ground lean beef
5 tablespoons crisp whole wheat
  bread crumbs
1 scant tablespoon tomato paste
2 teaspoons low-fat fromage blanc
  or yogurt
2 tablespoons grated Parmesan
  cheese

1 small onion, finely chopped
1 eggplant (¾ to 1 pound) baked,
  peeled, and coarsely chopped
  (see page 28)
1 to 2 cloves garlic, minced
Salt and freshly ground pepper to
  taste

1. Preheat the broiler to its highest temperature. Place the broiler shelf in its lowest position. Line the tray with foil, shiny side up. Place the broiler rack on the tray.

2. Thoroughly mix together all ingredients, reserving 2 tablespoons bread crumbs. Shape the mixture into 4 fat oval cakes. Dredge them, on both sides, in the reserved crumbs. They may be frozen at this point (see note below.)

3. Broil on the rack 4 inches from the heat source for 3 to 4 minutes on each side, until crusty on the outside and medium-rare within. (Cook more or less to your taste, but please don't incinerate them!)

4. Serve as they are, or in whole wheat buns with Browned Onions (page 16) and Red Pepper Sauce (page 161) or Red Pepper Ketchup (page 167). Or serve with a dollop of Creamy Pesto (page 160) on each burger.

  Prepare the eggplant in the microwave (page 28).

Note: To cook burgers from the frozen state, preheat the broiler, then broil approximately 2 inches from the heat for 5 to 7 minutes on each side.

SHEPHERD'S PIE

Serves 6 to 8

Shepherd's pie is one of the glories of traditional British home cooking. This particular pie is for a slim and healthy shepherd. Many changes can be rung on this familiar theme. See the suggestions below.

2 pounds lean ground lamb, or beef or veal	1 tablespoon low-sodium Worcestershire sauce
3 onions, finely chopped	2 tablespoons tomato paste
3 cloves garlic, minced	Salt and freshly ground pepper to taste
1¼ cups stock	Dash nutmeg
1¼ cups dry red wine	

About 5 cups well-seasoned
mashed potatoes (page 197)
made from 2 pounds potatoes
and ½ cup buttermilk

6 tablespoons grated Parmesan
cheese

1. Cook the ground lamb in a large, nonstick frying pan, breaking up the lumps as it cooks. When the lamb is cooked through, drain well in a colander. Spread it out on paper towels and blot with more paper towels. Wash and dry the frying pan. Return the drained and blotted lamb to the pan.

2. Meanwhile, combine onions, garlic, ¼ cup stock, and ¼ cup wine in a nonreactive frying pan. Simmer briskly, stirring occasionally, until the onions are tender and the liquid is almost gone. Add this mixture to the drained lamb.

3. Stir in the Worcestershire sauce, tomato paste, salt, and pepper. Stir in remaining stock and wine. Simmer, uncovered, for 20 to 30 minutes, stirring occasionally, until thick. Taste and adjust seasonings.

4. Spread the meat mixture in a gratin pan or in individual casseroles. Season the potatoes with nutmeg, and spread them over the meat. Sprinkle evenly with the Parmesan cheese. At this point the pie may be covered tightly with plastic wrap and refrigerated for up to 2 days. Bring to room temperature before proceeding.

5. Preheat the oven to 375 F. Bake the pie, uncovered, for 30 to 40 minutes, until browned and bubbly. Bake individual casseroles 20 to 30 minutes. Serve at once, or cool, wrap tightly, and freeze for a later meal. Reheat the unthawed frozen pie, covered, either in the oven or the microwave.

Variations:

What good is a classic if you can't fool around with it a bit? Here are some variations on the classic.

MEXICAN-STYLE SHEPHERD'S PIE

Use beef, pork, or a combination. When you cook the onions in step 2, add 1 tablespoon chili powder, 1 teaspoon crumbled dried oregano, ¼ teaspoon ground cinnamon, ½ teaspoon ground cumin, and ½ teaspoon crushed chiles. Omit the Worcestershire sauce in step 3. Season the mashed potatoes with a pinch or two of ground cumin and ground cayenne.

GREEK-STYLE SHEPHERD'S PIE

When you cook the onions in step 2, add 1 teaspoon cinnamon and ½ teaspoon crumbled oregano. Omit the Worcestershire sauce in step 3, but add the pulp of 1 baked eggplant (see page 28). Season the mashed potatoes with a pinch or two of cinnamon and some baked garlic purée (see page 25).

CURRIED SHEPHERD'S PIE

Serves 8

This is my all-time favorite shepherd's pie. I've made it many times and served it to the great and the near-great. Don't be afraid of the long list of ingredients—you are, basically, making your own curry powder with the long list of spices. The meat-eggplant mixture is at once hot, sweet, and sour, and the potatoes are creamy and mellow with the taste of baked garlic. This is a lean version of a recipe I originally published in my book *Potatoes* (Harmony).

2 large Spanish onions, coarsely
   chopped
1¼ cups stock
1 teaspoon turmeric
1 teaspoon cumin
1 teaspoon pure chili powder
1 teaspoon ground coriander

1 teaspoon ground cardamom
¼ teaspoon ground ginger
¼ teaspoon ground cinnamon
Pinch ground cloves, allspice, and
   nutmeg
Salt and freshly ground pepper to
   taste

3 cloves garlic, minced
1½ pounds lean ground lamb
Chopped pulp of 2 baked
  eggplants (page 28) (about ¾
  pound each)
One 14-ounce can chopped
  tomatoes
¼ cup raisins
4 tablespoons mango chutney
1 tablespoon fresh lemon juice
1 tablespoon Worcestershire
  sauce

8 dried apricot halves, minced
  (use scissors)
1 tablespoon tomato paste
Mashed potatoes made with 7
  large baking potatoes, salt,
  pepper, and 1 cup buttermilk
  (see page 197)
¼ teaspoon cayenne pepper
½ teaspoon garam masala
Purée from 1 head baked garlic
  (page 23)

1. Spread the onions out in a heavy frying pan. Add *no* liquid or fat. Heat the frying pan gently. Cook at moderate heat, without stirring, until the onions are sizzling and beginning to stick to the bottom of the pan.

2. Stir in the stock and let it bubble up, stirring up the browned bits in the pan as it bubbles. Stir in the spices and seasonings and the minced garlic. Reduce the heat and simmer, stirring frequently, until the mixture is very thick (not at all soupy) and the onions and spices are "frying" in their own juices. Don't rush this step; it is very important that the spices do not have a harsh, raw taste. Taste. Cook very gently for a few more minutes, if necessary. Scrape the mixture into a bowl.

3. In the same frying pan, cook the ground lamb over medium heat. As it browns, break up any lumps with a wooden spoon. When it is thoroughly cooked, drain very well in a colander set over a bowl. Discard the drained fat. Put the lamb and the onion mixture back into the frying pan.

4. Stir in the eggplant pulp, tomatoes, raisins, chutney, lemon juice, Worcestershire sauce, and apricots. Simmer for 30 minutes, stirring occasionally. Stir in the tomato paste and simmer for 5 to 10 minutes more, until thick. Taste and adjust seasonings. Spread the mixture into a gratin pan. Preheat oven to 375 F.

5. Season the potatoes with cayenne pepper, garam masala, baked garlic purée, and salt and pepper. Taste and add more seasoning, if needed. Spread the potatoes over the meat.

6. Bake for 40 to 50 minutes, until brown and bubbling.

KEEMA CURRY

Serves 6; makes 5½ cups

179 Calories per serving
1.6g fat
(Traditional keema curry: 448 Calories
per serving, 28.8g fat)

This is an Indian home-style dish that sticks to the ribs. Make sure that your ground beef is very lean. Keema reheats well from both the refrigerator and the freezer. In fact, it improves with time.

2 medium onions, cut into eighths
2½ cups stock
2 teaspoons minced fresh peeled
  ginger
2 cloves garlic, minced
1 teaspoon ground cinnamon
1 teaspoon ground coriander
Pinch ground cloves
½ teaspoon cayenne pepper
½ teaspoon ground allspice
6 whole green cardamom pods,
  lightly crushed

1 bay leaf, broken in half
1 fresh green chili, stemmed,
  seeded, and minced
2 medium boiling potatoes, cut
  into 1-inch cubes
3 tablespoons tomato paste
Salt and freshly ground pepper to
  taste
1½ pounds very lean ground beef
One 14-ounce can chopped
  tomatoes
1 teaspoon garam masala

1. Separate the segments of the onion pieces and spread them out in a heavy frying pan. Add *no* liquid or fat. Heat the frying pan gently. Cook at moderate heat, without stirring, for 7 to 10 minutes, until the onions are sizzling, speckled with dark amber, and beginning to stick to the pan.

2. Stir in half of the stock and let it bubble up, stirring up the browned bits in the pan with a wooden spoon as it bubbles. Stir in the ginger, garlic, spices, and chili. Reduce the heat a bit and simmer, stirring frequently, until the mixture is very thick (not at all soupy), and the onions and spices are "frying" in their own juices. Don't rush this step; it is essential that the spices should not have a raw, harsh taste. Taste. Cook very gently for a few more minutes, if necessary. Remove bay leaf.

3. Toss the potatoes in the spice mixture until they are well coated. Stir in the tomato paste. Season to taste.

4. In another frying pan, cook the meat until it loses its red color. Break it up with a wooden spoon as it cooks. Drain well in a colander. Spread out the meat on paper towels and blot with more paper towels to eliminate even more fat. Stir the meat into the onion-potato mixture.

5. Stir in the remaining stock and the tomatoes. Bring to a boil. Reduce heat and simmer briskly for about 30 minutes, uncovered, until the mixture is thick. Cover and simmer for 15 minutes more, until the potatoes are done. If at any time the mixture threatens to stick and burn, stir in a bit more stock. Stir in the garam masala. Serve with basmati rice and Cucumber Raita (page 203).

CHILI CON CARNE

Makes 5 cups

This is a great Texas chili, with one non-Texas aberration—a real Texan would never stir the beans in with the meat; he or she would eat them on the side. If you wish, add chopped, peeled red, green, and yellow peppers to the onions and spices in step 2. It's not traditional, but it's *good*.

2 large onions, coarsely chopped
About 2 cups stock
2 cloves garlic, crushed
2 tablespoons chili powder
1 teaspoon ground cumin
1 teaspoon dried oregano, crumbled
1 teaspoon crushed dried chili, optional (use depending on the strength of the chili powder and your taste)
1½ pounds very lean coarsely ground beef
4 tablespoons tomato paste
One 15-ounce can red kidney beans, rinsed and drained
Salt and freshly ground pepper to taste

1. Separate the segments of the onion pieces and spread them out in a heavy frying pan. Add *no* liquid or fat. Heat the frying pan gently.

Cook at moderate heat, without stirring, for 7 to 10 minutes, until the onions are sizzling, speckled with dark amber, and beginning to stick to the pan.

2. Stir in 1¼ cups stock and let it bubble up, stirring up the browned bits in the pan with a wooden spoon as it bubbles. Stir in the garlic and spices. Reduce the heat a bit and simmer, stirring frequently, until the mixture is very thick (not at all soupy), and the onions and spices are "frying" in their own juices. Don't rush this step; it is essential that the spices not have a raw, harsh taste. Taste. Cook very gently for a few more minutes, if necessary.

3. In another nonstick frying pan, cook the meat until it loses its red color. Break it up with a wooden spoon as it cooks. When the meat is thoroughly cooked, drain very well in a colander over a bowl. Spread out the meat on paper towels and blot with more paper towels to eliminate even more fat.

4. Combine the meat and the onion mixture. Stir in the tomato paste, beans, and enough remaining stock to just cover the contents of the pan. Add salt and pepper to taste. Bring to the simmer. Simmer, uncovered, until the mixture is thick, about 30 minutes.

ITALIAN MEAT SAUCE

Makes 4½ cups

Everyone loves meat sauce. This version stretches a small amount of meat into a sumptuous amount of sauce. It's good on all types of pasta. Consider unusual shapes as well as the standard ones. My assistant served the sauce with couscous, and it was a wonderful combination. And at a buffet I attended, the hostess dispensed with pasta altogether and served it on a bed of braised carrot slices. Brilliant!

½ pound very lean ground beef
1 medium onion, chopped
2 large cloves garlic, crushed
1 small red pepper, peeled,
    seeded, and chopped

1 small yellow pepper, peeled,
    seeded, and chopped
Two 1-pound cans chopped
    tomatoes

4 heaping tablespoons tomato paste	1 tablespoon chopped fresh basil, or ¼ teaspoon dried
One 2-inch piece of Parmesan cheese rind	½ pound button mushrooms, quartered
Salt and freshly ground pepper to taste	½ cup dry red wine
1 tablespoon chopped fresh oregano, or ¼ teaspoon dried	½ cup stock
	Several dashes low-sodium soy sauce

1. Cook the beef and onion in a heavy, nonstick frying pan over medium heat. As the meat browns, break up any lumps with a wooden spoon. When the meat is almost browned, stir in the garlic and peppers. Continue to stir and cook until the meat is completely cooked through and the onions are limp. Place the mixture in a colander over a bowl to drain away any fat. Spread it out on paper towels and blot with more paper towels. Return it to the frying pan.

2. Add the chopped tomatoes, tomato paste, Parmesan rind, salt, pepper, and herbs. Cover the frying pan and simmer for 15 minutes.

3. Meanwhile, put the mushrooms, wine, stock, and soy sauce into a nonreactive, nonstick heavy frying pan. Stir to combine everything very well. Simmer, stirring occasionally, until the liquid is almost gone. Let the mushrooms "fry" gently in their own juices for a few moments. Do not let them scorch or stick. Add the mushrooms to the sauce.

4. Season the sauce to taste and simmer, partially covered, for approximately 10 minutes more, until thick. The sauce may be refrigerated for a day or so, or frozen. Serve with pasta, or as a filling for baked potatoes.

OLD-FASHIONED BEEF STEW

Makes 10 cups

A good beef stew cannot be made with extra-lean meat. In the finished stew, cubes of such meat will be as dry as dust. Choose well-marbled slabs of chuck steak. This recipe shows you how to use the fat marbling in the meat to advantage. As the stew braises, the fat and the gelatin melt out of the meat, leaving it very tender. Then all of the fat rendered from the meat is meticulously removed, leaving a rich, but low-fat, gravy. I sent samples of this stew to a laboratory for analysis, to assure myself that the fat really was eliminated. Raw chuck braising steak contains 9.4 percent fat, the finished recipe had only 1.75 percent fat!

3 pounds very well trimmed chuck steak, cut into ¾-inch cubes
½ teaspoon dried thyme
1 bay leaf, crumbled
¼ cup brandy
2 cups red wine
2 cloves garlic, crushed
2 cups beef stock
3 carrots, scraped and sliced
3 onions, cut in half and sliced into thin half-moons

1 medium floury potato, peeled and cut into ½-inch dice (Idaho Russet potatoes work well here)
Salt and freshly ground pepper to taste
1 pound button mushrooms, quartered
½ cup chicken stock
1 tablespoon low-sodium soy sauce

1. Combine the beef, thyme, bay leaf, brandy, 1½ cups wine, and garlic in a plastic bag and close tightly. Allow to marinate for at least an hour, turning the bag occasionally. If you wish, refrigerate and leave overnight.

2. Preheat oven to 350 F.

3. Strain the marinade into a saucepan. Add the beef stock. Boil until reduced by about one-third. Skim off all foam and scum as it boils.

4. Combine the beef, marinade, carrots, onions, potato, salt, and pepper in a heavy, nonreactive casserole. Cover tightly and bake for 2 to 2½ hours, or until the beef is tender. Reduce the oven temperature as needed during the cooking time to maintain a gentle simmer. It must not boil.

5. Pour the stew into a sieve set over a large bowl. Cover the meat and vegetables well so that they do not dry out. Pour the juices into a glass jar and place in the freezer.

6. Put the mushrooms, ½ cup wine, chicken stock, and soy sauce in

a nonstick frying pan. Simmer until the mushrooms are almost tender and the liquid greatly reduced. Season to taste.

7. When the stew juices in the freezer are thoroughly chilled, the fat will have risen to the top and congealed on the surface. Scrape off and discard every bit of the fat. In the stew pot, combine the defatted juices and the mushrooms with their juice. Bring to a boil. Stir in the meat and vegetables. Simmer for a few minutes for the flavors to blend.

8. Mash a few of the potato pieces against the side of the pot and then stir. The crushed potatoes will thicken the stew. Taste and adjust the seasonings to your liking. The stew may be refrigerated for a day or two before serving. The flavor will improve.

BEEF IN RED WINE

Makes 6 cups

This is a simplified, low-fat, drastically Calorie-reduced version of *boeuf bourguignonne*.

3 large Spanish onions, chopped	3 pounds very well trimmed
2¼ cups chicken stock	chuck steak, cut in ¾-inch
¾ cup dry red wine	cubes
1 pound mushrooms, quartered	1 tablespoon tomato paste
Several dashes of low-sodium soy	Salt and freshly ground pepper to
sauce	taste
½ teaspoon dried thyme	6 cloves garlic, halved
½ teaspoon dried tarragon	

1. Preheat the oven to 350 F.

2. Combine onions and 1½ cups stock in a heavy nonreactive frying pan. Cover and boil for about 5 minutes. Uncover and simmer briskly until tender, browned, thick, and syrupy. Raise the heat, pour in ¼ cup wine and boil until the alcohol has evaporated and the onions are a deep amber-brown. Purée half the mixture. Combine the puréed and unpuréed mixtures. Set aside.

3. Combine the mushrooms, remaining ¾ cup stock, ½ cup wine, soy sauce, and herbs in a heavy nonreactive frying pan. Simmer briskly, stirring occasionally, until the mushrooms are tender and the liquid just about absorbed. Do not let the mushrooms scorch.

4. Combine the meat cubes with the mushrooms and onions in a baking dish. Add tomato paste, salt, and pepper, and stir so that everything is well combined. Bury the garlic pieces in the stew. Bake in the oven, covered, for 30 minutes. Reduce the heat to 300 F, and cook for another 2 to 2½ hours, or until the meat is very tender. Reduce the oven temperature, if necessary, to keep stew at a very gentle simmer.

5. Drain, saving the juices. Cover the meat well to prevent it from drying out. Chill the juices in the freezer until the fat rises to the top and hardens. Discard the fat. Recombine the meat and juices. Refrigerate or freeze until needed.

BEEFSTEAK ON A BED OF ONIONS WITH RED PEPPER SAUCE

Makes 8 pieces

Serve this to very special guests on a very special occasion. There is no need to babble about the low-Calorie and low-fat levels. If you don't tell, no one will have an inkling that this is diet food. The dish is easy if you are organized. Have the Red Pepper Sauce and the Browned Onions made in advance (they can be made several days, or even weeks, ahead of time and frozen). The last-minute preparation and cooking is then a snap.

8 center-cut filet mignon steaks, about ½ inch thick	½ cup dry red wine
Freshly ground pepper	1 recipe Red Pepper Sauce (page 161)
1 bunch trimmed scallions, sliced	1 recipe Browned Onions (page 16), heated to sizzling point
4 tablespoons chopped fresh parsley	

1. Preheat the oven to 200 F.

2. Trim the steaks of any vestige of fat. Trim them into neat rounds.

3. Spread a sheet of wax paper on your work surface. Sprinkle lavishly with freshly ground pepper. Place the steaks on the paper. Grind lots more pepper on top of the steaks. Cover with another sheet of wax paper. With a kitchen mallet, gently pound the meat.

4. Heat a nonstick frying pan until hot. Place the steaks in the pan so that they are not touching each other. (Do this in 2 batches, if necessary.) Cook over high heat on one side for 2 to 3 minutes. Turn and cook on the second side for 2 to 3 minutes. At this point the steaks will be nicely browned on the outside and juicy and pink within. Remove them with tongs to a platter and cover loosely with foil. Put them in the oven to keep warm.

5. Scrape the scallions and parsley into the frying pan and pour in the wine. Boil, stirring and scraping with a wooden spatula to loosen all the browned bits, until almost all the liquid is gone. Reduce heat and stir in the Red Pepper Sauce. Pour in any juices that have collected under the meat. Stir and cook for a few minutes.

6. Spread out the Browned Onions onto a warm platter. Overlap the steaks on the bed of onions. Pour a ribbon of pepper sauce down the length of the meat. Serve at once, passing the rest of the sauce in a gravy boat.

FLANK STEAK

What a remarkable cut of meat: extremely lean, deeply flavorful, economical, and—if you cook it rare or medium-rare—very tender. Broil or pan-sauté flank steak without fat. Let it rest for 5 to 10 minutes for the juices to redistribute, and then slice it thin, against the grain. Flank satisfies steak cravings without guilt, and because of the way it is served—sliced thin and lavished with sautéed mushrooms or onions or a Slim Cuisine sauce—a little goes a long way.

FIVE-SPICE STEAK

Serves 4 to 6

Five-spice powder is a fragrant Chinese mix of spices. Many super-markets now stock it, but if you can't find it make your own with equal parts of ground cinnamon, fennel, star anise, cloves, and ginger.

1 tablespoon coarsely chopped
  fresh ginger
4 large garlic cloves
1½ teaspoons five-spice powder
2 cups water
½ cup sherry
¼ cup low-sodium Worcestershire
  sauce

½ tablespoon sugar
1 strip orange zest (3 inches x 1
  inch)
1 flank steak (approximately 1
  pound), well trimmed

1. In a nonreactive pan, simmer all ingredients except the steak for 15 minutes. Let cool.

2. Put the steak in a shallow, nonreactive dish and pour the marinade over it. Marinate for several hours or overnight, turning occasionally.

3. Preheat the broiler to its highest setting. Remove the meat from the marinade, discarding the marinade. Cook the steak 3 inches from the heat for 4 to 5 minutes per side for rare; 6 to 7 minutes per side for medium-rare.

4. Let meat rest for 3 to 4 minutes. Slice thinly against the grain, and serve.

PEPPERED STEAK WITH MUSHROOM SAUCE

Serves 4 to 6

In this zesty preparation for flank steak, the mushroom sauce has echoes of both Mexico and New Orleans.

1 flank steak (approximately 1 pound), well trimmed
Freshly ground pepper to taste
Salt to taste
1 medium onion, finely chopped
1 small carrot, finely chopped
2 cloves garlic, minced
1 small stalk celery, finely chopped
One 4-ounce can mild green chiles, chopped (save the juices)
½ teaspoon dried oregano, crumbled
2 canned plum tomatoes, drained and chopped
1¼ cups stock
Dash low-sodium soy sauce
1 bay leaf
½ pound mushrooms, quartered
2 to 3 tablespoons chopped fresh parsley

1. Grind pepper over both sides of the meat and press it in. Let stand for 15 minutes.

2. Heat a heavy, nonstick frying pan until moderately hot. Sear the meat on both sides, using tongs to turn the meat.

3. Reduce the heat a bit and cook for 3 to 4 minutes on each side. Salt lightly on both sides. Remove to a warm platter, cover loosely with foil, and keep warm.

4. Add the onion, carrot, garlic, celery, chiles, 1 teaspoon chili juice, oregano, tomatoes, half the stock, soy sauce, bay leaf, and mushrooms to the pan. Boil, stirring and scraping the bottom of the pan, until the vegetables are tender and the liquid greatly reduced.

5. Return the meat and its accumulated juices to the pan and simmer, turning the beef with tongs as it cooks, for 1 to 2 minutes, to heat it through and cook it to your liking. To be tender the beef must remain rare or medium-rare.

6. Taste and adjust seasonings, adding a bit of salt if necessary or an extra dash of soy sauce. Discard the bay leaf. Slice the meat thinly

against the grain and arrange on a warm platter. Pour the sauce over it and serve at once.

Variations:

Sauté the steak (steps 1 to 3) until rare or medium-rare and then try one of the following:

STEAK AND MUSHROOMS

Serve the sautéed steak simply, with Sautéed Mushrooms (page 20). Sauté the mushrooms in the pan in which you have cooked the beef.

STEAK PIZZAIOLA

Serve the sautéed steak with Tomato Sauce (page 166).

STEAK WITH GARLIC-WINE SAUCE

When the steak has been sautéed, keep it warm. In the steak pan, boil 5 ounces each red wine and stock until reduced and syrupy. Add some thyme and tarragon, if you like. Stir in the purée of 1 head of baked garlic (see page 23). Season with salt and pepper. Slice the meat, and pour the sauce over it.

STEAK AND ONIONS

The eternal classic—serve the sautéed, sliced steak with Sweet-and Sour-Onions (page 19) or Browned Onions (page 16).

STUFFED FLANK STEAK

Serves 4

When sliced, a beautiful pinwheel of vivid green spinach is revealed. This is also good served cold or at room temperature, as well as warm. Leftovers are delicious in sandwiches, with a bit of the cold sauce spread on the bread.

2 cups dry red wine
Juice and grated rind of ½ lemon
¼ cup low-sodium Worcestershire
  sauce
1 bay leaf
4 cloves garlic, crushed
1 teaspoon grated fresh ginger

About 1 pound flank steak,
  trimmed of any fat
1½ pounds fresh spinach
Salt and freshly ground pepper to
  taste
1 large Spanish onion, cut in half
  and sliced into thin half-moons

1. Preheat oven to 475 F.

2. Combine red wine, lemon juice and rind, Worcestershire sauce, bay leaf, garlic, and ginger in a wide, shallow nonreactive dish.

3. Butterfly the steak as follows: Slit it down the long end with a very sharp knife; cut it very carefully almost all the way through until you can open it flat like a book. Or better yet, have the butcher do this for you.

4. Marinate the steak in the wine mixture while you prepare the spinach. Wash the spinach well, stem it, and tear it into shreds. Put it in a nonreactive saucepan and stir it over moderate heat, until limp but still bright green and fresh-tasting. (It will cook in the water clinging to its leaves.) Drain well. Stir in 3 tablespoons of the marinade.

5. Remove the steak from the marinade. Pour the marinade into a saucepan and boil until reduced by half.

6. Open out the flank steak. Spread the spinach over the surface to within 1 inch of the edges. Starting from a long edge, roll the beef like a jelly roll, into a long sausagelike shape. Tie the roll securely crosswise in several places with kitchen string.

7. Place the beef roll on a rack in a nonreactive baking pan that can be used on top of the stove as well as in the oven. Sprinkle it with a bit of salt, a generous amount of pepper, and the onion slices. Pour in the marinade. Roast for 10 minutes, turning it after the first 5 minutes.

8. Reduce the oven temperature to 350 F. Roast the meat for 20 minutes more, turning it halfway through the roasting time.

9. Remove the meat from oven. Put it on a platter, cover loosely with foil, and let it rest for 15 minutes. Leave the onions in the baking dish. Place the baking dish on top of the stove. Bring the pan juices to a boil. Boil until the liquid is dark brown, thick, and syrupy. Remove from the heat. Stir in any meat juices that have accumulated under the meat roll.

10. Remove and discard the string. Slice the meat thinly and serve, with the pan juices and the onion slices.

PORK MEDALLIONS ESTERHAZY

Serves 6

My version of the classic Hungarian dish is rich and filling, a perfect choice for a winter dinner party. The original royal Hungarian version was made with beef. If you wish, serve the sauce and vegetable garnish with lean filet mignon, cooked rare either under the broiler or in the pan (see page 118).

1 pork tenderloin (1 to 1¼ pounds), trimmed of all fat	Esterhazy Sauce (following recipe)
Salt and freshly ground pepper	Garnish (page 126)
1 cup stock	

1. Cut the pork into ¾-inch slices. Sprinkle with salt and pepper.

2. Heat a heavy, nonstick frying pan until moderately hot. Sear the pork slices for 1 to 2 minutes on each side, until browned (do not crowd them). Pour in the stock, simmer, turning frequently, for approximately 5 minutes, until cooked through and tender. Transfer to a plate, cover loosely with foil, and keep warm.

3. Boil the stock for a few seconds, scraping the bottom of the pan with a wooden spatula. When the stock is thick and syrupy, reduce the heat and return the pork slices to the pan. With tongs, turn them a few times.

4. Arrange the pork on a warm platter. Stir the syrupy stock into the Esterhazy Sauce. Pour some sauce over the pork. Top with the drained hot vegetable garnish. Serve at once. Pass the rest of the sauce in a gravy boat at the table.

ESTERHAZY SAUCE

Makes 2 cups

This is a most delicious sauce. Its richness is amazing, yet it contains virtually no fat. It may be made ahead of time and stored in the refrigerator. Bring to room temperature before proceeding with the recipe.

1 large onion, chopped
2 small carrots, scraped and
  chopped
2 small parsnips, peeled and
  chopped
2½ cups stock
1 bay leaf
Salt and freshly ground pepper to
  taste

Grated zest of 1 lemon
Juice of ½ lemon
1 tablespoon Dijon mustard
½ cup quark, or ½ cup
  "smoothed-out" drained low-fat
  cottage cheese mixed with 1 to
  2 ounces skim milk

1. Combine the vegetables with ½ cup stock in a heavy frying pan. Cover and simmer briskly for 4 to 5 minutes. Uncover and simmer until the vegetables are almost tender and the liquid just about gone.

2. Add the remaining stock, bay leaf, salt, pepper, lemon zest, and lemon juice. Let simmer gently, uncovered, until the vegetables are very tender. Discard the bay leaf. Cool slightly. Purée the mixture in a blender with the mustard and the quark or cottage cheese. Pour it into a saucepan.

3. Simmer gently for approximately 5 minutes. Taste and adjust seasonings. Remove from heat. Cover with a piece of plastic wrap directly over the surface of the sauce to prevent a skin from forming and set aside until needed.

♡ ☆ ◔ GARNISH FOR PORK ESTERHAZY

This is good enough to serve as a vegetable accompaniment to other dishes on occasion, or use to top fish fillets *en papillote* (see page 94).

1 parsnip
1 carrot
1 stalk celery

1 cup stock
Salt and freshly ground pepper to
    taste

1. Scrape the vegetables and cut them into julienne.
2. Combine the vegetables with the stock and simmer briskly, stirring constantly, until they're tender and the stock is thickened and reduced. Season to taste, and set aside until needed.

POULTRY

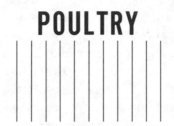

Chicken is famous for being low-fat and good for you, but it needs some help before it can live up to its reputation. Be ruthless with the chicken that you take home from the store. Pull off all the lumps of fat. Denude the bird of its fatty skin—all of it. Only then is the chicken ready for Slim Cuisine. The white meat is leaner than the dark, and each requires different handling.

Chicken Breasts

Skinless, boneless chicken breasts are perfect for a quick, elegant meal. When properly cooked, they have a remarkably creamy and delicate texture. If they are overcooked, however, they become stringy and dry. Many quality butchers and supermarkets carry chicken breasts from free-range birds that have been skinned, boned, and split. When you get them home, meticulously trim away any traces of fat, gristle, and skin. Under each chicken breast is a loose, narrow flap of flesh. Pull it off and save it for stir-fries or chicken salad. The trimmed deflapped chicken breast is called the *"suprême"* or the "cutlet." A 3½-ounce chicken cutlet contains negligible fat. It is an excellent source of protein. It can be quickly pan sautéed in a heavy nonstick frying pan and served with a delicate sauce. Sauté the chicken until it is just done, so that it is tender and plumply juicy.

Chicken Legs and Thighs

Unlike the breasts, the dark meat of chicken takes beautifully to slow, gentle braising. When cooked with flavorsome ingredients, the meat becomes succulent and comforting; perfect cold-weather fare. Before cooking the legs and thighs, remove and discard all skin and fat. For many braised dishes, consider cooking the dish the day before serving. Store it in the refrigerator. The next day, any fat in the sauce will have congealed. Spoon it out and discard it. Then reheat the casserole and serve. And remember that the meat from free-range birds is the most delicious.

♡ ◔   **PAN-SAUTÉED CHICKEN BREASTS**

Heat a heavy, nonstick frying pan until moderately hot. Season the chicken cutlets with salt and pepper. Cook for 3 minutes on the skinned side, then carefully turn and cook on the second side, for approximately 3 minutes, or until *just* cooked through (it will feel firm but a little springy when touched with your finger).

Chicken breasts prepared in this manner may be used with a variety of sauces, either hot or cold. Consider the following: Yellow Pepper Sauce (page 133), Red Pepper Sauce (page 161), Beet Purée (page 181), Esterhazy Sauce (page 125), Tomato Sauce (page 166), Rémoulade Sauce (page 66), Creamy Pesto (page 160). Or top the breasts with Sautéed Mushrooms (page 20) and shredded mozzarella cheese. Broil for 1 to 2 minutes, until the cheese is melted and bubbly.

CHICKEN-BERRY SALAD

♡ ⏲

Serves 6

This is the most elegant of chicken salads. Serve it as a main dish at a light supper or a special luncheon. With its berries, creamy-textured chicken breast, and light dressing, this salad is the essence of summer. Shredded poached chicken may be substituted for the chicken cutlets, or use smoked chicken.

6 chicken cutlets (see page 127)
1 pound mixed fresh berries
  (blueberries, blackberries,
  strawberries, raspberries)
½ pound red or green seedless
  grapes
8 ounces drained low-fat fromage
  blanc or yogurt

Juice of ½ small lemon
½ teaspoon mild honey
2 tablespoons buttermilk
Salt and freshly ground pepper to
  taste
Fresh mint leaves for garnish

1. Cook the chicken according to the pan-sauté method (see preceding recipe).
2. Slice each chicken cutlet into crosswise slices on the diagonal. Overlap them on a pretty platter. Surround the chicken with the mixed berries and grapes.
3. Combine remaining ingredients except the mint leaves. Pour a bit of dressing in a stripe down the center of the chicken slices. Garnish with the mint leaves. Serve the rest of the dressing separately.

MOLDED CHICKEN SALAD

♡

Makes 4 cups

This is lovely as a luncheon dish or as a first course for a special dinner party. It makes a good sandwich filling, too. Be sure that you season it well; it should not be bland.

Juice of 1 lemon
⅓ cup chopped chives
½ cup chopped fresh dill
½ cup chopped fresh parsley
½ cup yogurt or fromage blanc
  "Cream Cheese" (page 21)
1 cup buttermilk
Cayenne pepper to taste
1 large stalk celery, finely minced

2 poached 3-pound chickens (use
  the poached chicken left from
  making stock, page 31, or see
  recipe for quick Poached
  Chicken, page 144)
Salt and freshly ground pepper to
  taste
Watercress for garnish

1. In a bowl, combine lemon juice, herbs, yogurt cheese, 5 table-spoons buttermilk, cayenne pepper, and celery.

2. Pull the chicken from the bones in chunks and shred it finely with your fingers. As you shred each chunk, stir it into the bowl of dressing. Discard every bit of fat, skin, and gristle.

3. Stir in more buttermilk until the texture is creamy but not too loose. Season to taste with salt and freshly ground pepper and more cayenne, if desired. The flavor should be very lively.

4. Tightly pack the mixture into a 4-cup mold (heart-shaped is nice). Cover and refrigerate overnight. The mixture will taste quite yogurty at first, but it will mellow overnight until it tastes as if it were made with a lemony mayonnaise.

5. At serving time, loosen the molded chicken all around with a thin-bladed knife. Unmold it onto a pretty serving plate. Garnish with watercress and serve.

CURRIED CHICKEN SALAD

Makes 6 cups

This is an elegant, spicy version of the Molded Chicken Salad. It's a show-stopping buffet dish.

7 shallots, peeled and chopped
8 ounces golden raisins
½ cup chicken stock

½ cup raspberry vinegar
2 teaspoons minced fresh ginger
4 cloves garlic, minced

1 teaspoon turmeric
2 teaspoons each: ground cumin,
  ground coriander, ground
  cinnamon
¼ teaspoon ground cloves
½ teaspoon crushed dried chiles
½ teaspoon ground allspice
½ cup yogurt or fromage blanc
  "Cream Cheese" (page 21)

Approximately 1 cup buttermilk
½ cup chopped fresh parsley
1 large stalk celery, finely minced
2 poached chickens
Salt, freshly ground pepper, and
  cayenne pepper to taste
Fresh coriander sprigs for garnish

1. Spread the shallot pieces in a heavy frying pan. Add *no* liquid or fat. Heat the frying pan gently. Cook at moderate heat, without stirring, for 7 to 10 minutes, until the shallots are sizzling, speckled with dark amber, and beginning to stick to the pan.

2. Stir in the raisins, stock, and raspberry vinegar and let it bubble up, stirring up the browned bits in the pan with a wooden spoon as it bubbles. Stir in the ginger, garlic, and spices. Reduce the heat a bit and simmer, stirring frequently, until the mixture is very thick (not at all soupy) and the shallots and spices are "frying" in their own juices. Don't rush this step; it is essential that the spices should not have a raw, harsh taste. Taste. Cook very gently for a few more minutes, if necessary. Let cool.

3. In a large bowl, combine the cooled mixture with the yogurt "cream cheese," 5 tablespoons of buttermilk, the parsley, and celery.

4. Pull the chicken from the bones in chunks and shred each chunk into the bowl. Discard every bit of fat, skin, and gristle.

5. Stir in more buttermilk until the texture is creamy but not too loose. Season with salt, freshly ground pepper, and cayenne, if you want it very spicy. Tightly pack the mixture into a mold as described in the preceding recipe. Refrigerate overnight. At serving time, unmold it onto a pretty plate and garnish with fresh coriander sprigs.

OVEN-"FRIED" CHICKEN WITH MINT DIPPING SAUCE

Makes 8 pieces of chicken

130 Calories per leg
2.4g fat
(Traditional fried chicken: 232 Calories
per piece, 7.3g fat)

Oven-"frying" produces juicy, crispy-crusted chicken that is prepared without a speck of oil or fat. The dipping sauce is Indian-inspired.

1½ cups plain low-fat yogurt
1¼ cups bread crumbs
Salt and freshly ground pepper to taste

4 chicken thighs, skinned
4 chicken legs, skinned
Dipping Sauce (following recipe)

1. Preheat oven to 400 F.

2. Pour the yogurt into a wide, shallow bowl and set it on your work surface.

3. Season the bread crumbs with salt and pepper. Spread the crumbs out on a platter next to the yogurt.

4. Place a wire rack over a baking sheet and set aside.

5. Dry the chicken pieces. Dip each piece into the yogurt until thoroughly coated on both sides. Then roll each piece in the crumbs, pressing the piece in so that the crumbs adhere. Each piece should be evenly coated.

6. Place the chicken on a wire rack. Bake for 40 to 45 minutes, or until just done.

7. To serve, place a piece of chicken on each of 4 small plates. Pour some sauce in a crescent on the bottom edge of each plate, around the chicken but not on it. Put the remaining pieces of chicken on a platter and pass the remaining sauce in a clear glass pitcher.

Note: If you don't use dairy products with meat, dip the chicken into egg white instead of yogurt and choose a vegetable purée sauce (see index) instead of the following one.

DIPPING SAUCE

1½ cups plain low-fat yogurt
½ small onion, coarsely chopped
1 thin slice fresh ginger, peeled
  and chopped
1 teaspoon chopped fresh chiles,
  or more to taste

Salt to taste
6 tablespoons fresh mint leaves
2 tablespoons fresh coriander
  (Chinese parsley) leaves
2 tablespoons fresh parsley leaves

Place all the ingredients in a blender or food processor. Flick the motor on and off until a thin, green-flecked sauce is achieved. Serve at once with the chicken.

CHICKEN WITH YELLOW PEPPER SAUCE

Makes 4 pieces with 2 cups sauce

The rich, buttery-yellow pepper sauce complements the juicy chicken cutlet very well. You will find the sauce useful in many other ways as well.

½ cup dry white wine or dry
  vermouth
3 ounces tarragon wine vinegar
2 tablespoons minced shallots
½ teaspoon dried tarragon,
  crumbled
1 tablespoon chopped fresh
  parsley

Pinch of cayenne pepper
6 yellow bell peppers, seeded and
  coarsely diced
1¼ cups stock
Salt and freshly ground pepper to
  taste
4 chicken cutlets (see page 127)

1. Combine the first six ingredients in a small saucepan. Bring to a boil, reduce heat, and simmer briskly until almost all the liquid has evaporated. Set aside.

2. Combine the peppers and stock in a deep, heavy frying pan.

Bring to a boil. Cover, reduce heat, and simmer for 20 to 30 minutes, until tender. Let cool.

3. Purée the peppers in a blender or food processor. Strain through a sieve or strainer, rubbing the peppers through with a rubber spatula or a wooden spoon. The skins will be left behind. Discard them.

4. Put the purée in a saucepan. Simmer for a few minutes until it is thick enough to coat the back of a spoon. Stir in the tarragon infusion and season to taste with salt and pepper. This sauce may be prepared several days ahead and stored in the refrigerator until needed. Warm it while the chicken is cooking.

5. Heat a heavy, nonstick frying pan until moderately hot. Season the chicken with salt and pepper. Cook for 3 minutes on the skinned side, then carefully turn and cook on the second side for approximately 3 minutes or until *just* cooked through. (It will feel firm but a little springy when touched with your finger.) Place the chicken on a plate and cover loosely with foil.

6. Stir any juices that have accumulated under the chicken into the hot yellow pepper sauce. Ladle a generous amount of the sauce onto warm dinner plates. Slice each chicken cutlet crosswise into ½-inch slices. Overlap the slices from each cutlet on the puddle of sauce. Serve at once.

CHICKEN WITH RASPBERRIES

Makes 4 pieces

This is one of the most exciting chicken breast recipes I know. The garlic cloves are cooked and served like a vegetable. Use fresh, firm, unblemished bulbs. The manner of cooking ensures that they become tender and mild—not the slightest bit overpowering or "garlicky." If the thought of raspberries with garlic is just too shocking, omit the raspberry garnish (but not the raspberry juice—it is essential to the goodness of the sauce). Although you have to thaw a package of frozen raspberries to get the little bit of juice needed, you can make a batch of Raspberry Sauce (see page 229) with the thawed berries for use in a dessert later in the week.

16 large garlic cloves	Salt and freshly ground pepper to
1 teaspoon sugar	taste
3½ tablespoons raspberry vinegar	1 to 2 tablespoons raspberry juice
½ cup chicken stock	and a few raspberries for
4 chicken cutlets (see page 127)	garnish (see note)

1. Combine the garlic, sugar, 1½ teaspoons vinegar, and 1½ teaspoons water in a small saucepan. Bring to a boil. Reduce heat and simmer, uncovered, for about 3 minutes, until the sugar dissolves. Increase the heat to a rapid simmer, cover, and let cook until the garlic is tender and caramelized and the liquid is just about gone, about 10 minutes.

2. Add the stock and the remaining vinegar and boil, uncovered, for another minute. Set aside.

3. Heat a heavy, nonstick frying pan until moderately hot. Season the chicken with salt and pepper. Cook for 3 minutes on the skinned side, then carefully turn and cook on the second side for approximately 3 minutes, or until *just* cooked through. (The pieces will feel firm but a little springy when touched with your finger.) Place the chicken on a plate and cover loosely with foil.

4. Add the sauce and garlic to the frying pan. Bring to a boil, stirring and scraping with a wooden spoon as you do so. Add 1 to 2 tablespoons of juice from the thawed raspberries. After about a minute the sauce will be thick and syrupy. Remove from the heat. Taste and season with a tiny bit of salt and some pepper.

5. Pour any juices that have accumulated under the chicken into the sauce. Add the chicken and turn it to coat with the sauce. Arrange the chicken on a serving plate. Pour the sauce and the garlic over and around it. Garnish with berries. Serve at once.

Note: Use thawed frozen unsweetened raspberries to make the garnish. Some of the juice will be used in step 4 to augment the sauce.

CHICKEN CURRY

Serves 6

This is an exquisite dish, excellent served warm, tepid, or cool. It does not reheat well. The only tricky thing about the recipe is the timing. You want to catch the chicken at the exact moment of doneness, when it is creamy, tender, and perfect.

6 chicken cutlets, skinned and
  boned
Juice of 1 large lemon
Salt to taste
1 teaspoon each: ground turmeric,
  ground cumin, ground
  coriander
½ teaspoon each: sugar, crushed
  dried chiles, ground cinnamon

½ bay leaf, finely crumbled
2 cloves garlic, minced
2 medium onions, cut into eighths
1¾ cups stock
2 tablespoons tomato paste
3 tablespoons raisins
3 tablespoons plain low-fat
  yogurt, at room temperature

1. Cut the chicken cutlets crosswise into strips that are approximately 1 inch wide. Each cutlet will yield about 5 strips. Put the strips in a bowl, squeeze the lemon juice over them, sprinkle with a bit of salt, and toss with 2 spoons to combine. Set aside.

2. Place all the spices and herbs in a small bowl. Add the minced garlic.

3. Separate the segments of the onion pieces and spread them in a heavy frying pan. Add *no* liquid or fat. Heat the frying pan gently. Cook at moderate heat, without stirring, for 7 to 10 minutes, until the onions are sizzling, speckled with dark amber, and beginning to stick to the pan.

4. Stir in 1¼ cups stock and let it bubble up, stirring up the browned bits in the pan with a wooden spoon as it bubbles. Stir in the spices and garlic. Reduce the heat a bit and simmer, stirring frequently, until the mixture is very thick (not at all soupy) and the onions and spices are "frying" in their own juices. Don't rush this step; it is essential that the spices not have a raw, harsh taste. Taste and cook very gently for a few more minutes, if necessary.

5. Toss the chicken into the spicy onions in the frying pan. Stir and turn the chicken over low heat for 1 minute, until everything is well combined. Stir in ½ cup stock and the tomato paste and raisins. Spread the mixture out evenly in the pan. Cover and cook over the *lowest* heat for 4 minutes more.

6. Uncover. Add 2 tablespoons yogurt and stir over *low* heat for a few moments, until everything is combined. Stir in the last tablespoon yogurt and cook, stirring, for a moment or two more. Check the chicken for doneness. It should feel firm and springy, not soft and mushy. If you wish, cut into several pieces. You may even cut each strip in half. Each piece should be pearly white in the center. Try to catch them when they are *just* done, at the moment they are turning from blush pink to creamy white. A minute or two of overcooking turns them tough and stringy. If they are not done yet, replace the cover, turn off the heat and let them sit for a minute or two more. Stir everything once more, and serve warm or at room temperature.

CHICKEN IN ONION-TOMATO GRAVY

Makes 12 pieces

This homey chicken stew has an Indian accent. It is best made in advance so that the flavors mellow and the congealed fat can be removed the next day.

4 large onions, cut into eighths	Pinch ground cloves
2 cups stock	8 cardamom pods, lightly crushed
1 tablespoon minced peeled fresh ginger	1 bay leaf, broken in half
4 cloves garlic, minced	2 cinnamon sticks, broken in half
1 teaspoon ground cumin	Two 14-ounce cans crushed tomatoes
1 teaspoon ground coriander	6 chicken legs, skinned
¼ teaspoon cayenne pepper, or to taste	6 chicken thighs, skinned
	Salt and pepper to taste

1. Separate the segments of the onion pieces and spread them in a heavy, 12-inch frying pan. Add *no* liquid or fat. Heat the frying pan gently. Cook at moderate heat, without stirring, for 7 to 10 minutes, until the onions are sizzling, speckled with dark amber, and beginning to stick to the pan.

2. Stir in 1¼ cups stock and let it bubble up, stirring up the browned bits in the pan with a wooden spoon as it bubbles. Stir in the ginger, garlic, and spices. Reduce the heat a bit and simmer, stirring frequently, until the mixture is very thick (not at all soupy), and the onions and spices are "frying" in their own juices (about 15 minutes). Don't rush this step; it is essential that the spices not have a raw, harsh taste. Taste and cook very gently for a few more minutes, if necessary.

3. Stir the tomatoes into the onions. Set the pan aside.

4. Place the chicken thighs, skinned side down, in a nonstick frying pan. Heat gently until the chicken is sizzling. Do not add fat or oil! Brown the chicken thighs lightly, season with salt and pepper, turn and brown lightly on the other side (about 5 minutes per side). Blot them with paper towels, then place them, skin side down, in one layer, on the tomato mixture. Repeat with the chicken legs. Place them between and over the thighs. Blot the pan with paper towels in order to mop up the rendered fat.

5. Pour the remaining ¾ cup stock into the frying pan and boil rapidly, until it is reduced by more than half. Stir and scrape up the browned bits on the bottom of the frying pan as it boils. Pour the stock over the chicken.

6. Bring the tomato-chicken mixture to a boil. Reduce heat, cover, and simmer for 20 minutes.

7. At the end of 20 minutes, turn and rearrange the chicken pieces in the pan. Cover and simmer until the chicken is done, 20 to 30 minutes more.

8. Remove the chicken to a casserole or a platter. Cover loosely with foil so that it does not dry out. Tip the pan and skim as much fat as possible from the sauce. Boil the sauce for a few minutes, until it is thick and pulpy. Recombine the chicken and sauce, cover, cool somewhat, and refrigerate.

9. The next day, scrape out the congealed fat and discard it. Reheat the chicken and sauce gently before serving.

BRAISED HONEY-MUSTARD CHICKEN

Makes 12 pieces

Serve this with rice to soak up the mustardy juices.

1½ tablespoons honey
Juice of ½ lemon
2 cloves garlic, minced
½ teaspoon low-sodium soy sauce
1 to 2 pinches cayenne pepper
2 tablespoons Dijon mustard

6 chicken legs, skinned
6 chicken thighs, skinned
Salt and freshly ground pepper to
  taste
1 medium onion, coarsely
  chopped

1. Preheat the oven to 325 F.

2. In a small bowl, stir together the honey, lemon juice, garlic, soy sauce, cayenne pepper, and mustard.

3. Season the chicken with salt and pepper. Put the chicken and onions in a casserole. Pour and scrape the mustard mixture over the chicken. Mix together very well so that the chicken and onions are coated with the sauce. Cover the baking dish with foil so that no steam can escape.

4. Bake for 1½ hours. Serve with rice.

Note: This recipe can be made a day ahead of time and reheated—the flavor will improve. Cook the dish for only 1¼ hours on the first day, cool, and refrigerate. On the next day, scrape off any congealed fat, then reheat gently, covered, in the oven for 30 to 45 minutes.

CHICKEN BRAISED WITH GARLIC

Makes 12 pieces

78 Calories per piece
1.5g fat
(Traditional chicken braised with garlic:
166 Calories per piece, 2.8g fat)

This is my low-fat version of a famous French classic. *Everyone* loves this dish, even confirmed garlic haters. Slow, gentle cooking renders the usually pungent bulb sweet, mild, and mysterious.

40 cloves garlic (see note)
6 chicken legs, skinned
6 chicken thighs, skinned
2 medium onions, coarsely
  chopped
2 stalks celery, thinly sliced (save
  the leaves)
¼ cup chopped fresh parsley
1 teaspoon dried tarragon,
  crumbled

½ teaspoon allspice
¼ teaspoon cinnamon
Pinch cayenne pepper
Salt and freshly ground pepper to
  taste
¼ cup Cognac
3 ounces dry white vermouth

1. Preheat oven to 325 F.

2. Place all ingredients in a deep, heavy pot that can be covered. Combine everything very well with your hands. Seal the pot very tightly with foil. Place the pot cover over the foil. The pot must be very well sealed so that no juices or steam can escape.

3. Bake for 1½ hours, or until the chicken is very tender. Do not open the pot during this time.

4. Serve piping hot, with good crusty bread for mopping up the garlic and the juices. Open the pot at the table so that the diners get a blast of the wonderful fragrance that emerges as you open it.

Note: The garlic must be fresh and unblemished, with no shriveled cloves or green sprouts. If you wish, peel the garlic first by parboiling the cloves for 3 minutes in water to cover, then slipping off the skins. If you are in a rush, however, throw in the garlic unpeeled. As it cooks, it will become a purée within its skin. Encourage diners to squeeze the purée out of the skin with their forks and spread it on bread. Garlic haters can ignore it completely, although they will be missing something marvelous if they do. Have a few empty plates on the table to receive the discarded garlic husks and the gnawed chicken bones. This recipe can be made a day ahead of time and reheated—the flavor will improve. Cook the dish for only 1¼ hours on the first day, cool, and refrigerate. On the next day, scrape off the congealed fat, then reheat gently, covered, in the oven, for 30 to 45 minutes.

Variations:

Use the procedure in the preceding two recipes, but try these combinations of ingredients: Chicken Cacciatore—tomatoes, mushrooms, wine; Oreganato—lemon juice, oregano, onions, wine, garlic; Indian-Style—cardamom, cumin, coriander, cayenne, lemon juice and rind, onion, garlic, fresh coriander; American Barbecued—tomato purée, browned onions, cider vinegar, chiles, dash Worcestershire sauce, 1 to 2 pinches brown sugar.

CHICKEN VINDALOO

Makes 8 pieces

Indian vindaloos are sour and spicy, and beautifully pungent.

2 to 3 tiny chili peppers, thickly sliced
1 medium onion, cut into chunks
2 cloves garlic, lightly crushed
1 piece (2 inches long) fresh ginger, peeled and cut into chunks
1 teaspoon whole cumin seeds

1 teaspoon whole coriander seeds
1 teaspoon turmeric
1 teaspoon whole mustard seeds
2 tablespoons white vinegar
8 chicken legs, skin and fat removed
Salt to taste

1. Combine all the ingredients except the chicken and salt in the blender. Purée the mixture, stopping to scrape down the sides of the container with a rubber spatula.

2. Slash each chicken leg in 2 or 3 places with a sharp knife. Toss the chicken and spice paste together. Allow to marinate for at least 1 hour.

3. Gently heat a heavy, nonstick frying pan that can hold the chicken pieces in one layer. When moderately hot, put in the chicken pieces and spice paste. Cook gently for 1 to 2 minutes, turning the chicken with tongs, until it has just lost its raw look. Do not brown it.

4. Turn the heat to the lowest point. Salt the chicken lightly. Cover the pan tightly and cook for about 1 hour, or until the chicken is very tender, turning the chicken every 15 minutes or so.

CHICKEN BHUNA

Makes 8 pieces

Eat this vibrant Indian dish at once; it does not reheat well.

1 medium onion, chopped
1¼ cups stock
2 cloves garlic, minced
1 teaspoon peeled, chopped fresh ginger
1 teaspoon turmeric
½ teaspoon ground cinnamon
½ teaspoon freshly grated nutmeg
½ teaspoon ground allspice

1 teaspoon ground cumin
1 teaspoon chili powder
Pinch cloves
½ bay leaf, broken in half
2 to 3 tablespoons tomato paste
8 chicken thighs, skinned
Chopped fresh coriander for garnish

1. Spread the onion pieces in a heavy frying pan. Add *no* liquid or fat. Heat the frying pan gently. Cook at moderate heat, without stirring, for 7 to 10 minutes, until the onions are sizzling, speckled with dark amber, and beginning to stick to the pan.

2. Stir in the stock and let it bubble up, stirring up the browned bits in the pan with a wooden spoon as it bubbles. Stir in the garlic, ginger,

and spices. Reduce the heat a bit and simmer, stirring frequently, until the mixture is very thick (not at all soupy) and the onions and spices are "frying" in their own juices. Don't rush this step; it is essential that the spices should not have a raw, harsh taste. Taste and cook very gently for a few more minutes, if necessary.

3. Stir in the tomato paste. Add the chicken and stir it around to coat it thoroughly with the spice mixture.

4. Cover and cook over the lowest possible heat for about 1 hour, until the chicken is very tender. Turn the pieces occasionally. Discard the bay leaf pieces. Serve garnished with chopped coriander.

CHICKEN TARRAGON PIE

Serves 6

Here is a satisfying and interesting main course that uses both tender chicken meat and the Slim Cuisine Onion-Herb Infusion. It is a sort of souffléd, savory bread pudding. Serve with a salad of dark, leafy greens sprinkled with an interesting vinegar—balsamic, sherry, or raspberry. The more interesting the vinegar, the less you will miss the olive oil. Because it contains high-fat eggs, make this pie only occasionally. If you do not have a poached chicken on hand, use the quick Poached Chicken recipe (following recipe) or buy a ready-cooked roasted chicken from the supermarket. The pie also works beautifully with smoked chicken. Be sure to remove all skin and fat before using it.

6 ounces stale bread torn into chunks (5 cups)
1 recipe Onion-Herb Infusion, made with tarragon (page 17)
1 small poached or smoked chicken, shredded (about 3 cups)
2 ounces part-skim mozzarella cheese, shredded

2 tablespoons grated Parmesan cheese
3 tablespoons chopped fresh parsley
3 eggs
½ cup buttermilk
1½ cups skim milk
Freshly ground pepper and cayenne pepper to taste

1. Preheat the oven to 350 F.

2. In a bowl, toss together the bread, infusion, chicken, cheeses, and parsley. Spread this mixture in a 9-x-13-inch shallow glass or ceramic baking dish.

3. Beat the eggs with the buttermilk. Gradually beat in the skim milk. Season to taste with the peppers. You will probably need very little salt because the infusion, the Parmesan, and the peppers give plenty of flavor. Pour this mixture over the chicken-bread mixture. With a broad spatula or pancake turner, press the bread down into the liquid. Let stand for 1 hour in a cool place.

4. Bake for 40 to 45 minutes, until puffed and set. To test for doneness, insert a knife near the center—it should come out clean. Cut the pie into squares, and serve.

POACHED CHICKEN

If you want to poach a chicken in a hurry, use this nifty technique taught to me by a Chinese friend.

One 2½-pound chicken

1. Bring 6 quarts water to a boil in a deep pot.

2. Pull all excess fat from the chicken and wash it well, inside and out, in cold water. Submerge the chicken in the boiling water. When the water returns to a full boil, cover, and boil hard for 12 minutes (5 minutes per pound).

3. Remove the pot from the heat and let the chicken cool in the pot. (Do not leave it to cool at room temperature for more than 2 hours. It can, however, be refrigerated overnight, pot, cooking liquid, and all.)

4. Remove it from the liquid. (It will still be quite warm so be careful.) Remove the skin. Pull the meat off the bones in large pieces. Discard all tendons and gristle. Tear the meat into chunks, or shred

it. Refrigerate in a shallow dish, moistened with a bit of stock and well covered with plastic wrap until needed. This chicken is lovely in chicken salad, or try it in Chilaquiles (following recipe).

CHILAQUILES

Serves 6

This is an exciting, unusual, and splendid recipe: a low-fat version of authentic Mexican home cooking. There are many versions, but they always involve layers of corn tortilla pieces and piquant sauce. Sometimes meat or, as here, chicken is layered in, too. The original versions are swimming in fat. I have used the recipe successfully (and spectacularly!) with smoked chicken, and if you are in a hurry you might want to use a ready-cooked roasted chicken from the supermarket. Just be sure that you remove all skin and fat before using it. Corn tortillas are available in cans or frozen or refrigerated in many supermarkets and specialty shops. Reduce the amount of chili peppers if you don't like spicy food.

1 large onion, chopped
2½ cups chicken stock
1 medium fresh chili pepper, seeded and coarsely diced
4 jalapeños canned in vinegar, drained and coarsely diced
Two 1-pound cans chopped tomatoes
2 cloves garlic
Salt to taste

5 corn tortillas, baked in a 300 F oven until crisp, then broken into pieces (see page 218)
Meat from one 2- to 2½-pound poached chicken (see Basic Chicken Stock, page 31, or quick Poached Chicken, preceding recipe), shredded
6 ounces part-skim mozzarella cheese, shredded (1½ cups)

1. In a heavy, nonreactive frying pan, combine the onion in ½ cup stock, cover, and bring to a boil. Reduce heat and simmer for 5 minutes. Uncover, raise heat and simmer very briskly, until almost all liquid has boiled away. Reduce heat and simmer gently, until the liquid

has gone and the onions are beginning to stick. Stir until they begin to toast and brown. Pour in a splash of stock and boil, stirring and scraping the browned bits on the bottom of the pan. Remove from the heat.

2. Place the fresh chili, jalapeños, tomatoes, and garlic in the blender. Blend to a smooth purée. Pour into the frying pan with the onions. Cook over low heat, stirring for a few minutes.

3. Add the remaining stock and salt to taste. Simmer, uncovered, for 25 to 35 minutes, until thick and pungent. At this point the sauce is almost hot enough to melt the frying pan. When it is mixed with the remaining ingredients, however, its piquancy will be somewhat diluted.

4. Preheat the oven to 350 F.

5. Layer one-third of the tortilla pieces, one-third of the sauce, one-third of the shredded chicken, and one-third of the cheese in a shallow nonreactive gratin dish or baking dish. Layer on the second third of tortilla pieces, sauce, chicken, and cheese. Layer on the remaining tortilla pieces, sauce, chicken, and cheese.

6. Bake, uncovered, for 35 minutes, until bubbly. Serve at once.

🕐🖴 Prepare the tortillas in the microwave (page 218) and use a store-bought cooked chicken (remove all fat and skin).

LEMON-ROASTED CHICKEN

Serves 4

This was inspired by a winning recipe in the London *Daily Mail*'s Slim Cuisine recipe contest. I don't know which is better, the moist chicken meat or the incredible gravy. Leftovers make superb sandwiches.

Juice of 1½ lemons
1 teaspoon black pepper
2 teaspoons ground cumin
1 teaspoon paprika or paprika
  paste

One 3-pound roasting chicken,
  trimmed of fat
½ to ¾ cup dry white wine

1. Mix the lemon juice with all the ingredients except the chicken and wine. Make small incisions all over the chicken (except in the breast) and rub in the lemon mixture. Loosen the breast skin and rub the lemon mixture under the skin. Place the squeezed lemon halves in the chicken's cavity. Marinate overnight.

2. Next day, preheat the oven to 450 F. Place a rack across a flame-proof shallow roasting pan. Place chicken on the rack and roast, breast down, for 15 minutes, breast up for approximately 45 minutes, until just done.

3. Allow the chicken to rest on a plate, loosely covered with foil. Tilt the roasting pan and prop it in the tilted position. With a large spoon, spoon out all fat (there will be plenty) and discard. Put the roasting pan right on the burner, and turn the heat on high. Stir and scrape up the drippings and browned bits. Pour in ½ to ¾ cup dry white wine. Boil, stirring and scraping, until you have a dark, thick, rich sauce, and the alcohol has cooked away. Discard skin and carve chicken. Serve this powerful juice with the carved chicken.

VEGETARIAN

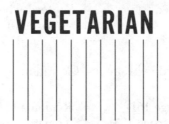

A meal does not always have to be focused on meat, poultry, or fish. Vegetables can easily be the star of a meal. There are vegetable recipes in other sections of the book as well that can be served as vegetarian main courses. Check the pasta and potato side-dish sections in particular.

VEGETARIAN FONDUE

This is one of my favorite meals, for guests as well as just family. It's colorful, fun, and unusual. Add protein by serving a starter that contains quark, yogurt cheese, fromage blanc, fish, et cetera (see the "Starters" chapter for ideas), or end with one of the buttermilk-based ice creams in the "Desserts" chapter. Choose your vegetables according to the season, and cook them carefully so that they are just done—flabby, mushy vegetables are unlovely things. Steaming is the best way to achieve perfection, both from a nutritional and culinary standpoint.

A selection of fresh vegetables, each steamed (or otherwise cooked) until done. Consider:

Cauliflower florets	Snow pea pods
New potatoes, unpeeled	Asparagus, peeled and trimmed
Broccoli florets	Zucchini, cut into sticks
Small turnips, quartered	Sautéed whole button mushrooms
French green beans	(page 20)

A selection of hot and cold sauces. Consider:

Red Pepper Sauce (page 161)	Rémoulade Sauce (page 66)
Yellow Pepper Sauce (page 133)	Tomato Sauce (page 166)
Beet Purée (page 181)	Creamy Pesto (page 160)

If you decide you'd like to add meat, choose a meatball recipe (see pages 99–107) and offer some as part of the selection. Arrange everything with color, texture, and shape in mind and, if you have small chafing dishes, use them to keep the warm sauces up to temperature. This is a convivial feast, perfect for a special celebration with good friends. If you have a microwave, you may facilitate the preparation by steaming the vegetables in advance. Let them cool, and then arrange them beautifully on individual plates. Cover tightly with plastic wrap. At serving time, microwave each plate to heat the vegetables through. Do not let them overcook, however.

♡ ☆   Serve the fondue without the creamy pesto.

GRILLED VEGETABLE LASAGNA

ɷ   Serves 4

Zucchini and eggplant sliced and grilled under the broiler are superb. The smokiness of the vegetables and the deep round taste of the tomato sauce combine to make a very satisfying lasagna.

1 eggplant, sliced crosswise, ¼
  inch thick
4 to 5 zucchini, sliced crosswise,
  ¼ inch thick
8 ounces quark or "smoothed-
  out" drained low-fat cottage
  cheese
6 ounces part-skim shredded
  mozzarella cheese
6 tablespoons grated Parmesan
  cheese

2 tablespoons skim milk
2½ cups chunky Tomato Sauce
  (page 166)
Salt and freshly ground pepper to
  taste
2 tablespoons mixed fresh herbs,
  such as basil and parsley
6 lasagna noodles, cooked *al
  dente* according to package
  directions

1. Preheat broiler at highest setting.

2. Spread eggplant slices in one layer on a nonstick baking sheet. Broil, close to the heat, for 5 to 7 minutes, or until lightly browned. (There is no need to turn them.) Cut each slice in half and set aside.

3. Spread the zucchini slices in one layer on a nonstick baking sheet. Broil, close to the heat, for 3 to 5 minutes, until speckled with brown. Set aside.

4. Preheat oven to 350 F.

5. Mix together the quark or "smoothed-out" drained cottage cheese with 3 ounces mozzarella, 3 tablespoons Parmesan, and the skim milk.

6. Spread 1¼ cups tomato sauce on the bottom of an 8-inch-square baking dish. Add a sprinkling of salt and pepper. Sprinkle 1 tablespoon of the mixed herbs over the sauce. Arrange 3 lasagna noodles on top. Place half the broiled eggplant slices on the noodles. Follow this with a layer of half the broiled zucchini slices, then all of the cheese mixture.

7. Spread the remaining tomato sauce over the cheese mixture, then a sprinkling of pepper, followed by the remaining mixed herbs. Arrange the remaining 3 lasagna noodles on top, followed by a layer of alternate rows of the remaining eggplant and zucchini. Sprinkle the remaining mozzarella and Parmesan cheese over the top.

8. Bake the lasagna for 40 to 50 minutes, until bubbling. Let stand for 5 to 10 minutes, then cut into squares and serve.

FARMER'S OMELETTE

Serves 4

Eggs are low in calories, full of high-quality protein and a fine collection of vitamins and minerals, but the yolks are, alas, high fat. One egg, once in a while, won't hurt, but don't make a habit of it. Save this for an *occasional* special weekend breakfast. But if you have high blood cholesterol, or a family history of high cholesterol and heart disease, then forget the omelette.

1 large baking potato, unpeeled, coarsely diced
1 large onion, chopped
3 cloves garlic, crushed
¾ to 1 cup stock
¼ cup red wine (optional)
3 eggs

1 egg white
2 to 3 tablespoons chopped parsley
Freshly ground pepper to taste
2 tablespoons grated Parmesan cheese

1. Combine the potato, onion, garlic, and stock in a frying pan. Bring to a boil, cover, and boil for 5 minutes.
2. Uncover, reduce heat, and simmer until the stock is almost gone and the vegetables are tender and beginning to brown. Pour in 1 ounce or so of wine or a splash of stock. Stir and scrape up the browned bits. Transfer the mixture to a large, *nonstick* omelette pan.
3. Preheat the broiler. Beat the eggs and the egg white with parsley, freshly ground pepper, and Parmesan cheese. Pour the egg mixture over the potato mixture. Let cook over medium heat without stirring for a few seconds, until the eggs begin to set on the bottom.
4. With a flexible plastic spatula, lift the edges of the omelette away from the pan, and tilt the pan so that the uncooked egg flows beneath the cooked portion. Continue doing this all around the pan until the omelette is almost completely set, but soft and runny in the center.
5. Place under the broiler for 2 to 3 minutes to set and very lightly brown the top. Serve at once, in wedges, straight from the omelette pan.

RAJMAA—RED KIDNEY BEANS

 Makes 5 cups; serves 8

This dish is adapted from a family recipe of Shashi Rattan. However, I have substituted the Slim Cuisine curry technique for her traditional one.

2 large onions, coarsely chopped
2½ cups vegetable stock
2 teaspoons minced fresh ginger
1 clove garlic, crushed
½ teaspoon ground cumin
½ teaspoon ground cinnamon
½ teaspoon ground coriander
Dash each ground cloves and
   cayenne
1 bay leaf

4 green cardamom pods, lightly
   crushed
One 1-pound-12-ounce can
   tomatoes
Two 15-ounce cans kidney beans,
   well rinsed and drained
Salt to taste
Chopped fresh coriander for
   garnish (optional)

1. Separate the segments of the onion pieces and spread them in a heavy frying pan. Add *no* liquid or fat. Heat the frying pan gently. Cook at moderate heat, without stirring, for 7 to 10 minutes, until the onions are sizzling, speckled with dark amber, and beginning to stick to the pan.

2. Stir in 1¼ cups stock and let it bubble up, stirring up the browned bits in the pan with a wooden spoon as it bubbles. Stir in the ginger, garlic, and spices. Reduce the heat a bit and simmer, stirring frequently, until the mixture is very thick (not at all soupy), and the onions and spices are "frying" in their own juices. Don't rush this step; it is essential that the spices should not have a raw, harsh taste. Taste and cook very gently for a few more minutes, if necessary.

3. Crush the tomatoes with your hands and add them with their juice to the onions. Simmer for 3 to 4 minutes.

4. Add the beans, salt, and remaining stock and simmer briskly for 15 to 20 minutes, until thick and savory. Taste and adjust the seasonings. Remove bay leaf. Serve garnished with chopped coriander, if desired.

PASTA AND SAUCES

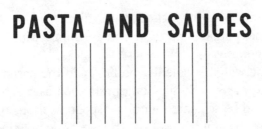

Slurping in the spaghetti (we never called it "pasta" in those days) was one of the few gastronomic glories of my childhood. The long, luscious strands were inevitably buried under unsophisticated oceans of tomato sauce and there were always some meatballs along to round things out nicely. Thinking of those comforting, sloppy meals of long ago makes me mistily nostalgic and ravenously hungry.

Here, to assuage both physical and psychic hungers, are grown-up versions of those fondly remembered spaghetti feasts. Fat and Calories have been drastically cut, and ingredients and techniques have been upgraded to match the hard-won sophistication of adulthood, but these dishes still satisfy me (as they will you) in those cozy dim recesses of the soul that only *spaghetti* can reach.

Pasta Guidelines

For the sake of nutrient density, choose whole-grain pastas occasionally. In specialty shops and supermarkets, there is a gorgeous array of shapes and sizes from tiny wheels and shells to long, ribbonlike *tagliatelle* and flat, broad lasagna. If you grew up on white pasta and suspect that the whole wheat variety is pure stodge, you are in for a pleasant surprise. It is delicate in both taste and texture and its gentle brown color is a lovely contrast to the brilliantly hued sauces into which it will be nestled. Cooking pasta perfectly is easy if you know the rules:

1. Bring plenty of lightly salted water to a rolling boil; at least 3½ quarts water per pound of pasta. If you are stingy with the water, the pasta will be gummy.

2. When the water is violently boiling, add the pasta, stirring with a wooden spoon as you do so. Long pasta such as spaghetti, linguini, et cetera, should be separated with the spoon as it begins to cook.

3. Stir frequently as it boils so that the pieces do not clump together. Never put the lid on the pot!

4. Do not overcook your pasta or you will end up with mush. Cook it until it is *al dente* (to the tooth). In other words, the pasta should be slightly resistant to the bite. Not at all raw, of course, but not at all mushy either. Begin fishing out pieces to taste—test early enough to avoid overcooking. (Use the timing suggested on the package as a guideline only.)

5. Have a large colander waiting in the sink. When the pasta is *just* done, don't dawdle. Use pot holders and extreme care. Drain it quickly into the colander, combine it with its sauce, and serve *at once*.

PASTA SHELLS ALFREDO

Serves 4 to 5

284 Calories per serving
2.6g fat
(Traditional pasta Alfredo: 707 Calories
per serving, 30g fat)

Here is an example of the Calorie savings made possible by substituting low-fat dairy products. This comforting dish is normally made with large quantities of butter and cream. You will find the Slim Cuisine version of this comfort food just as delicious and even more comforting than the original. (You have the extra comfort of knowing that you are not consuming too much fat.) This recipe may be multiplied or reduced as needed.

10 ounces pasta shells, or *tagliatelle* or fettuccine	¼ cup skim milk, at room temperature
8 ounces skim-milk quark or "smoothed-out" drained cottage cheese, at room temperature	3 tablespoons freshly grated Parmesan cheese
	Freshly ground pepper (optional)

1. Cook the pasta until it is *al dente*.

2. Meanwhile, scrape the quark or "smoothed-out" drained cottage cheese into a large warm bowl. With a wooden spoon, beat in the skim milk and grated Parmesan.

3. Drain the pasta, and immediately toss it into the cheese mixture. Grind in some pepper, if desired, and serve at once.

Elegant Variation:

Add baked garlic purée (see page 25) and a handful of chopped fresh herbs (chives, parsley, basil).

LASAGNA

 Serves 4 to 6

The tastiest lasagna is made with a meat sauce that is based on crumbled Italian sausage meat. The sausage is a combination of pork shoulder, aniseed, and crushed chiles. It's delicious but very high in fat. Here I have eliminated the high fat level, but kept the unique Italian sausage taste.

1 recipe Italian Meat Sauce (page 114)	eggplants, peeled, seeded (if the seeds are large), and
3 small (½ pound each) baked	chopped (see page 28)

½ to 1 tablespoon aniseed or
fennel seeds
1 to 2 good pinches crushed dried
chiles
1 pound low-fat quark or
"smoothed-out" drained
cottage cheese
4 ounces part-skim mozzarella
cheese, shredded

5 ounces skim milk
10 tablespoons grated Parmesan
cheese
5 ounces green or white lasagna
noodles, cooked *al dente*
according to package directions

1. Make the meat sauce, adding the chopped flesh of the eggplants, the aniseeds, and the crushed chiles before simmering the sauce. It should be well seasoned.

2. In a bowl, stir together the quark or "smoothed-out" drained cottage cheese, mozzarella, skim milk, and 7 tablespoons Parmesan.

3. Preheat the oven to 400 F.

4. Place a single layer of lasagna noodles in a baking dish (9 inches square, 2½ inches deep).

5. Cover with one-third of the meat sauce. Spread half the cheese mixture over the sauce. Spread an even layer of lasagna noodles over the cheese.

6. Repeat, making another layer of sauce, cheese, and lasagna.

7. Top with the remaining sauce and an even sprinkling of the remaining Parmesan.

8. Place a baking sheet on the oven floor to catch splatters and ease cleaning up. Bake the lasagna, uncovered, in the lower half of the oven for 45 minutes to 1 hour. Let stand for 15 minutes before cutting into squares, and serve. This freezes well.

CHICKEN LASAGNA

Serves 4 to 6

I love the spice-and-herb combination in this dish: allspice, tarragon, and a hint of soy sauce. Chicken Lasagna is delicious with a chicken that you poach yourself, a ready-cooked roasted chicken from the supermarket, or a smoked chicken.

5 bell peppers (mixed yellow and green), peeled, seeded, and chopped (see page 179)
3 medium onions, finely chopped
2 cloves garlic, minced
1 pound mushrooms, quartered
2½ cups stock
½ cup dry white wine
2 dashes low-sodium soy sauce
½ teaspoon allspice
½ teaspoon dried tarragon
Freshly ground pepper to taste
2 tablespoons tomato paste
Shredded or diced meat from 1 small (2- to 2½-pound) poached

or smoked chicken, all fat, gristle, and skin removed and discarded
1 pound skim-milk quark or "smoothed-out" drained cottage cheese
3 ounces part-skim mozzarella cheese, shredded
5 tablespoons grated Parmesan cheese
½ cup skim milk
7 ounces lasagna noodles, cooked *al dente* according to package instructions

1. Preheat oven to 400 F. Combine peppers, onion, garlic, mushrooms, 1 cup stock, wine, soy sauce, allspice, tarragon, and pepper in a large, nonstick frying pan. Stir to combine very well. Bring to a boil. Simmer briskly until the vegetables are tender and the liquid is greatly reduced and syrupy. Reduce the heat a bit and cook gently, stirring occasionally, while the vegetables "fry" in their own juices.

2. When the mixture is very thick and not at all soupy, stir in the tomato paste. Remove from the heat and stir in the chicken. Taste and adjust the seasonings. Set aside.

3. Stir together the quark or "smoothed-out" drained cottage cheese, mozzarella, 3 tablespoons Parmesan, and the skim milk. Set aside.

4. Choose a shallow, nonreactive 9-inch-square baking dish.

5. Put an even layer of lasagna noodles in the baking dish. Cover with half the chicken mixture.

6. Put an even layer of lasagna noodles over the chicken mixture. Cover with half the cheese mixture.

7. Put more noodles in an even layer over the cheese. Spread the remaining chicken mixture over it, then the remaining cheese mixture on top, mixing it in with the chicken mixture as you spread. Sprinkle 2 tablespoons grated Parmesan evenly over the top.

8. Bake at 400 F, for 45 minutes, until browned and bubbly and almost all the liquid is absorbed. Put the baking dish on a rack and let it sit for 15 minutes before cutting and serving.

Note: The lasagna may be refrigerated for several days or frozen. If desired, cut it into serving pieces and freeze in small microwave dishes, covered in plastic wrap. At serving time, pierce the plastic wrap in several places and microwave on full power for 4 minutes.

CREAMY PESTO

Makes 1¾ cups

27 Calories per tablespoon
1–2g fat
(Traditional pesto: 93 Calories per
tablespoon, 9g fat)

Pesto is a vividly colored and flavored thick Italian basil sauce, almost a paste. This version is made with quark or "smoothed-out" drained cottage cheese and roasted garlic purée. It is very good served tossed into hot pasta. Traditionally, pesto is made with plenty of olive oil. I have eliminated the oil altogether, and it tastes even better.

2 cups torn fresh basil leaves
1¼ cups roughly chopped fresh
  parsley
5 tablespoons freshly grated
  Parmesan cheese
1 ounce pine nuts *(pignoli)*
8 ounces quark or "smoothed-

out" drained low-fat cottage
  cheese
Purée from 1 to 2 heads baked
  garlic (page 23)
Salt and freshly ground pepper to
  taste

Combine all ingredients in the container of a food processor. Process to a thick paste. Scrape into a bowl and refrigerate. If your quark is very fresh to begin with, the sauce will keep for a week.

Note: If fresh basil is unavailable, do not substitute dried. Make Parsley Pesto, Dill Pesto, or Spinach Pesto by substituting any of those greens for basil. If you use dill, omit the Parmesan. Creamy Dill Pesto is the perfect accompaniment to cold poached salmon.

Suggestions for Serving Pesto

1. Fill Poached Mushroom Caps (page 57) with pesto. Arrange on juicy ripe sliced summer tomatoes. Garnish with whole basil leaves.
2. Toss the pesto with linguini, fettuccine, or penne. Serve with Sautéed Veal Meatballs (page 100) or Italian Sausage Balls (page 105).
3. Toss fettuccine or linguini with both pesto and Tomato Sauce (page 166). Add Sautéed Mushrooms (page 20), if you wish.
4. Serve pesto with slices of smoked salmon or spread on smoked salmon sandwiches.
5. Serve pasta with Italian Meat Sauce (page 114). Put a good dollop of pesto on top of each serving.

RED PEPPER SAUCE

 Makes 3¾ cups

This is a rich, thick, crimson pasta sauce with a vivid and lively taste. It packs a large flavor wallop with only 5 Calories per tablespoon! In addition to pasta, the sauce is lovely with steamed vegetables. For each serving, spoon some of the hot sauce in the center of a white or clear glass plate. Surround with a neat mound of vegetables that have been steamed until they are crisp-tender. Try peeled, trimmed asparagus, cauliflower florets, trimmed scallions, or green beans. To turn this combination into a hearty main dish, add broiled meatballs (page 99). If you want a smoky taste, grill the peppers (page 27) instead of simmering them in stock.

10 large red bell peppers, coarsely chopped
1½ cups stock
Salt, freshly ground black pepper, and cayenne pepper to taste

Onion-Herb Infusion, using thyme, basil, or tarragon (page 17)

1. Combine the peppers and stock in a deep, heavy frying pan. Bring to a boil. Cover, reduce heat, and simmer for 20 to 30 minutes, until tender.

2. Season with salt and black and cayenne pepper. Cool.

3. Purée the mixture in a blender or food processor. Strain through a sieve or strainer, rubbing it through with a rubber spatula or wooden spoon. The skins, which are tough, will be left behind. Discard them.

4. Put the purée into a saucepan. Stir in the infusion and simmer for 30 minutes. Taste and adjust seasoning. This sauce will keep in the refrigerator for a week.

Variation:

♡ ☆ ❆   **TOMATO-PEPPER SAUCE**

Combine Red Pepper Sauce with Tomato Sauce (page 166).

HELEN'S TERRACOTTA SAUCE

♡ ☆ ❆   *Makes 2½ cups*

I developed this sauce while my godson, Natty Bumpo, was staying with us. He and Helen Bray, his beloved nanny, helped to taste-test it. The color is a warm terracotta, the texture rough and chunky, and the taste rich. Serve it with pasta, fish, pan-sautéed chicken, or steamed cauliflower.

1 pound mushrooms, quartered	5 ounces dry white wine
2 onions, chopped	2 dashes low-sodium soy sauce
2 large red bell peppers, chopped	½ teaspoon dried tarragon
2 cloves garlic, crushed	½ teaspoon allspice
1 large carrot, scraped and	2 tablespoons tomato paste
coarsely grated	Salt and freshly ground pepper to
1 cup vegetable stock	taste

1. Combine the mushrooms, onions, bell peppers, garlic, carrot, stock, wine, soy sauce, tarragon, and allspice in a large nonstick frying pan. Stir to combine very well. Bring to a boil, reduce heat somewhat, and simmer briskly until the vegetables are tender and the liquid is greatly reduced and syrupy. Lower the heat and let the vegetables "fry" in their own juices, stirring occasionally.

2. Stir in the tomato paste. Season with salt and pepper. Cool slightly.

3. Purée the mixture in a blender or food processor. Push half of the purée through a nonreactive sieve. Combine the sieved and unsieved mixtures. Refrigerate until needed.

4. To reheat, pour into a saucepan and thin with 2 to 3 tablespoons stock or water. Simmer gently, stirring occasionally. Be very careful because the sauce is thick and is prone to violent, volcanic bubbling.

Pasta Pronto

Pasta suppers are fun. They provide plenty of scope for exuberant improvisation and they can often be prepared in less than 30 minutes. When you have worked late and are ready for a sumptuous and comforting meal, although you haven't had the time to plan for it, think of pasta. Put the water on to boil and choose your pasta type from the selection you are sure to have in the pantry. Then open the refrigerator and explore. Some of the most fascinating pasta sauces are born of a good leftover search. My favorite? Leftover Chili Con Carne (page 113), Tomato Sauce (page 166), and Sautéed Mushrooms (page 20) combined in a saucepan with a handful of raisins and a few pine nuts. Let it simmer gently while the pasta cooks (penne works well). When the penne is done, toss with the improvised sauce and, presto!, Pasta al Picadillo.

PENNE WITH PESTO AND SMOKED CHICKEN

Makes 10 cups

I invented this pasta dish for my mother-in-law when she came to visit. It was such a success that I made it again for my assistant's birthday lunch. Save this for very special occasions—it's glorious.

½ pound large mushrooms, cut into chunks

1 large red or yellow bell pepper, peeled, seeded, and cut into pieces (page 179)

1 onion, chopped

3 cloves garlic, chopped

¾ cup dry red wine

¾ cup stock

1 or 2 dashes low-sodium soy sauce

One 14-ounce can chopped tomatoes

1 piece Parmesan cheese rind

¼ teaspoon each: dried thyme, dried oregano, dried basil

1 tablespoon tomato paste

Salt and freshly ground pepper to taste

1 pound penne or *pennoni* (tubular, quill-shaped pasta)

8 ounces snow peas, fresh or frozen and thawed, destrung

4 to 6 ounces smoked chicken, cut into ½-inch cubes

½ cup Slim Cuisine Creamy Pesto (page 160)

1. Preheat the oven to its lowest setting. Put a large serving bowl in the oven to warm.
2. Combine the mushrooms, bell pepper, onion, garlic, wine, stock, and soy sauce in a heavy, nonreactive frying pan. Simmer briskly, stir-

ring occasionally, until the vegetables are tender and the liquid is thick and syrupy.

3. Stir in the tomatoes, Parmesan rind, herbs, tomato paste, salt, and pepper. Simmer gently, uncovered, for 15 minutes. Stir occasionally.

4. Meanwhile, cook the penne or *pennoni* in plenty of boiling salted water until *al dente.*

5. While the pasta is cooking, put the snow peas into a sieve or strainer. Just before the pasta is done, dip the sieve with the snow peas into the boiling pasta water. If the snow peas are frozen and thawed, leave in the boiling water for 2 seconds; if fresh for 10 seconds.

6. Drain the pasta in a colander. Pour it into the warm bowl. Immediately toss in the snow peas and the chicken. Toss with 2 spoons so that everything is well mixed. Remove the Parmesan rind from the sauce and stir the sauce into the pasta, tossing well to distribute it. Add the pesto, tossing so that everything is very well combined. Serve at once.

LEMONY PASTA SHELLS

                                  Serves 1

When you want to whip up something in a hurry that is satisfying yet low-Calorie, try this soothing pasta pilaf. (Broken-up angel hair pasta can be substituted for the shells, occasionally, for a change.) This amount makes a happy culinary indulgence for one, but you may satisfy a companion or two, as well, by doubling or tripling the recipe. As a variation, try adding garlic purée from roasted garlic to the infusion. For a more substantial dish, add Sautéed Veal Meatballs (page 100) before the final simmering. (The meatball version is a great family pleaser.)

1 recipe Onion-Herb Infusion (page 17)	1¼ cups boiling stock
2 ounces tiny pasta shells	Freshly ground pepper to taste
	Fresh lemon juice to taste

1. Heat the infusion in a pot. Toss the pasta with the infusion until it is well combined.

2. Stir in 1 cup hot stock and grind in some pepper. Cover and simmer over very low heat for 10 to 12 minutes, or until the liquid is almost absorbed. (It will be just a bit soupy.) If the pasta is still not done, add more stock, cover, and simmer until it is almost absorbed and the pasta is tender.

3. Squeeze in the lemon juice (I like to use the juice of 1 small lemon), stir, and serve at once.

TOMATO SAUCE

♡ ☆ ◔ ❉

Makes 3¾ cups

19 Calories per ½-cup serving
0.0g fat
(Traditional tomato sauce: 156 Calories
per serving, 7.7g fat)

If you think it is impossible to make a good tomato sauce without olive oil or butter, think again! This is fast, easy to make, and lovely on pasta, or pizza. Sautéed chopped red and yellow bell peppers and Sautéed Mushrooms (page 20) may be added. It freezes very well.

3 shallots, finely chopped
2 cloves garlic, peeled and
   crushed
Pinch cayenne pepper
¾ cup stock
¾ cup dry red wine, white wine,
   or vermouth
1 tablespoon chopped fresh
   parsley

1 tablespoon each chopped fresh
   basil, thyme, and oregano, or ¼
   teaspoon each dried
Four 14-ounce cans tomatoes,
   drained and crushed
Parmesan cheese rind
Salt and freshly ground pepper to
   taste
2 tablespoons tomato paste

1. Combine shallots, garlic, cayenne, stock, wine, and herbs in a heavy frying pan. Bring to a boil, reduce heat, and simmer briskly until almost all the liquid has been evaporated. Season to taste.

2. Stir in the drained tomatoes (you may crush them with your hands), Parmesan rind, salt, and pepper. Simmer, partially covered, for 15 minutes. Stir in the tomato paste and simmer 5 minutes more. Taste and adjust seasonings. Discard the Parmesan rind. Serve with pasta or on pizza, or try it spooned into baked potatoes.

Variation:

♡ ☆ ◔ ❄ SHAWM'S SMOOTH TOMATO SAUCE

My son loves homemade tomato sauce but hates lumps in his food. Should you have such a family member or friend, cool this sauce somewhat, then purée it in the blender. For a really smooth texture, rub the puréed sauce through a nonreactive sieve. It's convenient to make this sauce in bulk, and then store it in small containers in the freezer.

RED PEPPER KETCHUP

Makes about 3 cups

Use this thick, crimson, utterly splendid sweet-and-sour sauce to blanket your Slim Cuisine Hamburgers (page 107). And don't forget the "Sautéed" Onions (page 15)!

10 large red bell peppers, coarsely chopped
1¼ cups stock
Salt, freshly ground black pepper, and cayenne pepper to taste
Onion-Herb Infusion, using thyme, basil, or tarragon, or a combination (page 17)

3 tablespoons tomato paste
1 tablespoon brown sugar
½ teaspoon low-sodium teriyaki sauce
1 teaspoon low-sodium Worcestershire sauce
½ teaspoon rice wine vinegar

1. Combine the peppers and stock in a deep, heavy frying pan. Bring to a boil. Cover, reduce heat, and simmer for 20 to 30 minutes, until tender.

2. Season with salt, black pepper, and cayenne. Let cool.

3. Purée the mixture in a blender or food processor. Strain the purée through a sieve or strainer, rubbing it through with a rubber spatula or wooden spoon. The skins, which are tough, will be left behind. Discard them.

4. Put the purée into a saucepan. Stir in the infusion and the tomato paste, brown sugar, teriyaki sauce, Worcestershire sauce, and vinegar. Simmer, uncovered, for approximately 30 minutes, stirring occasionally until thick.

HERBED EGGPLANT SAUCE

Makes 2½ cups

A hearty, spicy sauce that is particularly good tossed with penne, ziti, or rotelli.

2 eggplants (about ½ pound each) baked (see page 28)
5 shallots, peeled, halved, and thinly sliced
½ to 1 tablespoon fennel seeds
1 tablespoon fresh or dried rosemary, crumbled
1 teaspoon crushed dried chiles, or to taste
½ cup dry red wine
1¼ cups chicken or vegetable stock

4 bell peppers (2 yellow and 2 red), peeled and cut into thin strips (see page 179)
One 14-ounce can chopped Italian tomatoes
1 to 2 tablespoons baked garlic purée (see page 25)
1 tablespoon tomato paste
Salt and freshly ground pepper to taste
1 piece Parmesan rind

1. Peel the baked eggplants and cut them in half. Discard any seeds that seem large and tough. Chop the flesh coarsely. Set aside.

2. In a frying pan, combine the shallots, fennel seeds, rosemary,

chiles, wine, and ½ cup stock. Boil briskly, stirring frequently, until almost dry. Add this mixture to the eggplant.

3. Heat ¼ cup stock in the frying pan in which you cooked the shallot mixture. When very hot, toss in the peppers. Stir-"fry" until the liquid is almost gone. Scrape the peppers into the eggplant mixture.

4. Combine with the remaining ingredients, including the remaining stock. Simmer for 10 to 15 minutes, until thick and savory. Taste and adjust seasonings. Serve with pasta or as a filling for baked potatoes or Potato Cases (page 191), or use as a filling in a vegetarian lasagna.

Microwave the garlic and eggplant, and use jarred peppers.

More Pasta Ideas

For a quick and delicious meal try any of the following tossed with the pasta of your choice.

- ⊕ ♡ Any vegetable (or combination of several vegetables) trimmed, cut up, and stir-"fried" in a combination of stock and wine. Add chopped herbs and some Slim Cuisine Sautéed Onions (page 15), if you wish.

- ⊕ ♡ Sautéed Mushrooms (page 20), alone or sautéed with peeled chopped yellow and red peppers and onions.

- ♡ Tzatziki (page 63).

- ⊕ ♡ Room-temperature yogurt mixed with salt and pepper and chopped fresh herbs. Add a clove or two of crushed garlic marinated in a bit of white wine vinegar, if desired.

- ⊕ ♡ Room-temperature "smoothed-out" low-fat cottage cheese or quark thinned a bit with skim milk, seasoned with ground cinnamon, caraway seeds, or poppy seeds. If desired, add some thinly sliced cabbage stir-"fried" in stock until just barely tender.

♡ Hummus (page 66).

♡ Salsa (page 188).

🕐 ♡ Tomato Sauce (page 166) to which you have added drained, flaked tuna in water, crushed raw garlic or baked Garlic Purée (page 25), a few capers, and a handful of chopped parsley. Add a dash or two of Tabasco sauce.

🕐 ♡ Tomato Sauce in which you have simmered stock-sautéed slivered carrots, cooked kidney beans, chick-peas, and chopped parsley.

♡ Browned Onions (page 16) and Stir-"Fried" Yellow and Red Peppers (page 179).

🕐 ♡ Mustard Cream (page 189).

♡ Creamy Pesto (page 160), Tomato Sauce, Italian Sweet-and-Sour Zucchini (see page 176), and Sautéed Mushrooms.

VEGETABLE SIDE DISHES

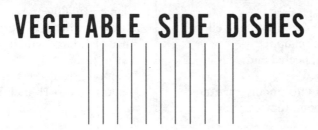

Steam your vegetables, sauté them, stir-"fry," bake, or braise them, but *please* don't boil them to death. Boiling robs them of many nutrients and causes small children to protest when presented with a plate of the miserably flabby things. What a glorious profusion of vegetables can be found in American farmers' markets as the seasons change. From the humble roots to slim, elegant asparagus, from familiar string beans to exotic fennel, from celery to celery root—experiment, taste, revel in the variety.

VEGETABLE CURRY

                    Makes 8¾ cups

This curry packs lots of nutrition into a very low-calorie, low-fat dish. The sauce is a thick and rich purée of onions, peppers, mushrooms, and carrots. Serve the curry with Cucumber Raita (page 203) and basmati rice for a delicious main dish, or serve it as part of an array of curries. I have also served it tossed into pasta.

2 large onions, cut into eighths	1½ teaspoons ground cumin
About 2½ cups stock	1½ teaspoons ground coriander
2 cloves garlic, crushed	½ teaspoon allspice

½ teaspoon ground turmeric
½ teaspoon ground ginger
¼ teaspoon cayenne pepper (to taste)
1 small red and 1 small yellow pepper, chopped
3 carrots, peeled and coarsely chopped
¾ pound mushrooms, quartered
1 tablespoon tomato paste

2 medium boiling potatoes, peeled and cut into 1½-inch dice
1 large cauliflower, trimmed and broken into large florets
Juice of ½ large lemon
Salt to taste
½ pound green beans, trimmed and cut into 1½-inch lengths

1. Separate the onion pieces into segments and spread them in a heavy frying pan. Add *no* liquid or fat. Heat the frying pan gently. Cook at moderate heat, without stirring, for 7 to 10 minutes, until the onions are sizzling, speckled with dark amber, and beginning to stick to the pan.

2. Stir in 1¼ cups stock and let it bubble up, stirring up the browned bits in the pan with a wooden spoon as it bubbles. Stir in the garlic, spices, peppers, carrots, and mushrooms. Reduce the heat a bit and simmer, stirring frequently, until the mixture is very thick (not at all soupy), and the vegetables and spices are "frying" in their own juices. Don't rush this step; it is essential that the spices should not have a raw, harsh taste. Cook very gently for a few more minutes. Stir in the tomato paste.

3. Cool slightly, then purée half the mixture in a blender and push it through a sieve. Combine the puréed and unpuréed mixture in the pan.

4. Add the potatoes and cauliflower to the pan. Toss everything together very well. Pour in additional stock to reach about one-third of the way up the sides of the pan. Squeeze the lemon juice over the contents of the pan. Season with salt. Bring to a boil.

5. Reduce heat, cover, and simmer for 15 minutes. Stir in beans and continue simmering for 5 minutes more, or until all the vegetables are tender.

Note: This reheats very well. If you plan to cook it ahead, undercook the curry slightly so that the vegetables do not turn to mush when they are reheated.

BRAISED CAULIFLOWER WITH FENNEL SEEDS

 Serves 4

This is a vegetable dish with enough interesting play of flavors to make it the star of a meal. It can be served hot or cold, but I like it best at room temperature, when all the splendid flavor seems to explode in the mouth. In order to improve its appearance, line a bowl with curly lettuce leaves, spoon in the cauliflower, then garnish with parsley.

1 large clove garlic, peeled
½ cup fresh parsley
1 tablespoon fresh or dried
   rosemary leaves
½ to 1 tablespoon fennel seeds
1¼ cups Browned Onions (page
   16) or Sautéed Onions (page
   15)
2 tablespoons balsamic vinegar

1 large or 2 small heads
   cauliflower, broken into florets
¾ cup stock
1 heaping tablespoon tomato
   paste
Salt and freshly ground pepper to
   taste
Chopped fresh parsley for garnish

1. Chop together the garlic, parsley, rosemary, and fennel seeds. Set aside.

2. Place the cooked onions in a deep, heavy frying pan. Heat until the onions begin to sizzle and stick to the frying pan. Pour in the vinegar and boil, stirring and scraping up the browned bits with a wooden spoon.

3. When the liquid is almost gone, stir in the garlic mixture. Add the cauliflower. Toss everything together until it is well combined.

4. Whisk together the stock and the tomato paste. Season with salt and pepper. Pour this mixture over the cauliflower and stir again. Bring to a boil, cover, reduce heat, and simmer until the cauliflower is very tender but not disintegrating (about 30 minutes in all). Cool to room temperature and serve, garnished liberally with chopped parsley.

Note: This may be prepared 1 to 2 days ahead, in fact the flavor will improve. Store it in the refrigerator. Bring to room temperature before serving. Add the parsley garnish just before serving.

GRATIN OF BAKED VEGETABLES

 Serves 4

Warming, comforting, and an attractive, glowing orange, this gratin freezes very well, and, when frozen, reheats beautifully in the microwave.

5 white turnips, peeled (about 1 pound)
6 medium carrots, scraped (about 1 pound)
Purée from one head baked garlic (see page 23)

2 to 3 tablespoons buttermilk
Salt and freshly ground pepper to taste
4 tablespoons freshly grated Parmesan cheese

1. Preheat the oven to 425 F.
2. Loosely wrap the whole turnips in foil, shiny side in, crimping the package well so that no steam escapes. Wrap the carrots in a similar fashion. Bake for 1 hour in the preheated oven, until the vegetables are very tender.
3. Unwrap. Trim stem and root ends. Place the turnips in a bowl and mash them with a potato masher. Scrape them into the bowl of a food processor. Cut the trimmed carrots into chunks, and add them to the turnips. Add the garlic purée.
4. Process the vegetables until they are smooth. Add the buttermilk and process until blended. Season to taste.
5. Scrape the mixture into a small, nonreactive gratin dish or shallow baking dish. Smooth the top and sprinkle with Parmesan. (The dish may be prepared ahead of time to this point. Refrigerate, well covered, until needed. It will keep for up to 2 days. Bring to room temperature before proceeding.)

6. Reduce the oven temperature to 350 F. Bake, uncovered, for 30 to 45 minutes, until browned on top and thoroughly hot.

♡ ☆   Omit Parmesan cheese.

Variations:

Parsnips or rutabagas may be substituted for the carrots or turnips. Potatoes may be added, although with potatoes, do not use a food processor. Purée by pushing them through a sieve or a food mill. Seasonings may be varied as well. Try ground allspice, cinnamon, cumin, or mace.

STIR-"FRIED" ZUCCHINI WITH LIME AND CUMIN

♡ ☆ ◔ ❋   *Serves 6*

This recipe is a prime example of how to stir-"fry," without oil. Try leftovers served cold with a sprinkling of interesting wine vinegar.

6 to 8 small zucchini	Generous pinch of ground cumin
½ cup stock	Juice of 1 to 2 limes
Freshly ground pepper to taste	Salt to taste

1. Wash and trim the zucchini but do not peel them. Cut them in half and then into strips about 2 inches long and ½ inch wide.

2. Pour the stock into a heavy, nonreactive frying pan. Bring to a boil.

3. Add the zucchini. Grind in a generous amount of pepper, and sprinkle in the cumin. With 2 wooden spoons, constantly toss and turn the vegetables over high heat, until they are crisp-tender and the stock has cooked down to almost nothing. Squeeze in the lime juice, season lightly with salt to taste, and let the zucchini stir-"fry" for a minute or so in their own juices. Serve at once.

Variations:

STIR-"FRIED" ZUCCHINI
♡ ☆ ◔ ❋   WITH GARLIC AND GINGER

Mince a clove of garlic and a thin slice of peeled fresh ginger. Put them in the frying pan with the stock and 1 fluid ounce dry sherry, and let boil for a few seconds before adding the zucchini. Omit the pepper and the lime juice. If desired, sprinkle with some chopped fresh coriander before serving.

STIR-"FRIED" ITALIAN
SWEET-AND-SOUR
◔ ❋   ZUCCHINI

Add 3 cloves garlic, minced, to the stock and let boil for a few seconds. Add the zucchini, freshly ground pepper, 2 tablespoons each raisins, rinsed and drained capers, and pine nuts, and the juice of 1 lemon. Just before serving, stir in some finely chopped parsley. Serve hot or cold.

♡ ☆   Omit the raisins and pine nuts.

STIR-"FRIED" CAULIFLOWER

♡ ☆ ◷ ✳   *Serves 4*

Cauliflower is very good steamed until crisp-tender. It is even better stir-"fried" in stock.

1 large head cauliflower	1 clove garlic, minced (optional)
¾ cup stock	Salt and freshly ground pepper to
Dash fresh lemon juice	taste

1. Cut off and discard the tough end of the cauliflower stalk. Discard the leaves. Separate the cauliflower in florets.
2. Pour the stock and lemon juice into a heavy wide nonreactive frying pan or wok. Heat to simmering. Toss in the cauliflower, optional garlic, and salt and pepper, cover, and simmer for 3 minutes.
3. Uncover. Raise the heat to high. Stir and toss the florets in the boiling stock until the stock is almost gone and the cauliflower is crisp-tender. Serve at once.

♡ ☆   # STEAMED ASPARAGUS

Please take the time to peel your asparagus before cooking it—what a difference it makes! This asparagus is so good that, in season, I often eat a large platter for dinner all by itself. If you want to get fancy, serve this asparagus as a first course with Red or Yellow Pepper Sauce (pages 161 and 133). Put a puddle of the sauce on a pretty plate, and surround the puddle with the beautiful green stalks. For a main course, add Sautéed Veal Meatballs (page 100).

Fresh asparagus stalks, washed

1. Cut off the tough woody bottom portion of each stalk. With a swivel-bladed vegetable peeler, peel each stalk from the bottom up to

the buds. If you are not going to cook them at once, stand them in a glass of water, as if they were a bunch of flowers.

2. Place the stalks in a steamer basket. Steam over boiling water for 3 to 7 minutes (depending on size) until crisp-tender. To test, pull out one stalk with tongs. Hold it up. It should just bend a *little* bit.

🕐 Use thin asparagus; it needs no peeling.

♡ ☆ # STIR-"FRIED" ASPARAGUS

Fresh asparagus stalks, washed
½ cup stock
Juice of ½ lime
Pinch fresh or dried thyme and
  tarragon

Salt and freshly ground pepper to
  taste

1. Trim and peel the asparagus (see preceding recipe), and cut them into 1-inch lengths. Heat the stock in a nonreactive wok or frying pan. Add the asparagus and toss and turn in the hot stock for about 2 minutes (use 2 wooden spoons or spatulas).

2. Squeeze in the lime juice, add a pinch each of thyme and tarragon, and salt and freshly ground pepper to taste. Keep stir-frying for a few more moments, until crisp-tender (more crisp than tender). Serve at once.

🕐 Use thin asparagus; it needs no peeling.

STIR-"FRIED" YELLOW
♡ ☆ ❄   **AND RED PEPPERS**

Peeling the peppers sounds tedious, but it is not much more difficult than peeling a carrot, and the textural difference between a peeled and unpeeled pepper is a big one. Without the skin, the peppers, when cooked in stock, produce a thick and delicious sauce. They are much more digestible when peeled, too. This is a very rich-tasting, colorful, and soul-satisfying vegetable dish, well worth the peeling time. Eat it as a vegetable accompaniment, try it tossed into pasta, or serve it as a sauce with flank steak (page 119) or Pan-Sautéed Chicken Breasts (page 128).

3 red bell peppers	**About 1 cup stock**
3 yellow bell peppers	**Freshly ground pepper to taste**

1. Cut the peppers in half, lengthwise. Remove the stem, seeds, and ribs. Cut the halves into their natural sections.
2. Peel each pepper piece with a swivel-bladed vegetable peeler. Cut each piece into strips about ½ inch wide.
3. Heat the stock in a heavy frying pan. When very hot, toss in the peppers and grind in some black pepper. With 2 wooden spoons, toss and turn the peppers in the hot stock until the liquid has cooked down considerably. Reduce the heat a bit and "fry" the peppers for a few minutes in their own juices, until they are very tender and the juices have formed a thick sauce. If necessary, add a bit more stock during the cooking. Serve the peppers at once with their delicious juices, or serve them at room temperature. This dish may be made in advance and rewarmed later or the next day.

CREAMED SPINACH

Serves 2 to 4

4 ounces low-fat quark or
  "smoothed-out" drained
  cottage cheese, at room
  temperature
2 to 3 tablespoons skim milk, at
  room temperature
Purée from 1 head baked garlic
  (page 23)

Salt and pepper to taste
Pinch nutmeg
1 pound spinach, very well
  washed, stemmed, and torn
  into strips

1. Stir together the quark or cottage cheese and milk. Stir in the garlic purée, salt, pepper, and nutmeg.

2. Put the spinach into a large, nonreactive pot. Cook, stirring, in the water that clings to its leaves, until limp and greatly reduced in volume but still bright green. Drain in a colander.

3. Fold the spinach and the quark mixture together. Serve at once.

🕐 🔲 Buy prewashed spinach. Bake garlic in the microwave.

 # BAKED BEETS

Make the most of beets by baking them. No other cooking method brings out their sweetness and flavor as well, and the texture will be very good indeed. Trim the greens away (save them to steam and serve like spinach—superb!) and wrap the whole, unpeeled beets in heavy-duty foil, shiny side in (3 to 4 beets may go in 1 package). Bake at 400 F for 1 to 2 hours, until tender. (Timing depends on age and size of the beets.) Use a skewer to test doneness. The skewer should go in easily, but the beets should not be mushy. Cool, then trim and slip off the skins. Serve sliced with a sauce of 2 to 3 parts yogurt to one part Dijon mustard (less mustard if you don't like spicy food)

mixed with a clove of crushed garlic that has marinated for a few minutes in a little bit of wine vinegar. Season with salt, freshly ground pepper, and 1 or 2 pinches sugar.

🕐 ▣ *To microwave large beets:*

Trim the beets and wrap each in microwave-safe plastic wrap. Microwave at full power for 15 minutes (1 beet) or 20 minutes (6 beets). Turn them over and microwave for another 15 minutes (1 beet) or 20 minutes (2 beets).

BEET PURÉE

                     Makes 2½ cups

Ruby red and textural, this is an unusual and interesting purée. Serve it mounded in Poached Button Mushrooms (page 57) or spoon dollops onto the wide ends of endive leaves. Or serve it as a spread on black bread, with smoked salmon if you're feeling luxurious. The mushroom and endive versions make a visually stunning party dish, especially if they are arranged on a black plate. I like to keep this purée for snacking; it makes a dandy between-meal nibble.

2 pounds baked beets (page 180), or use ready-cooked beets from the supermarket (if they are very vinegary, omit the vinegar)
8 tablespoons low-fat fromage blanc or yogurt or "smoothed-out" drained cottage cheese

1 to 2 cloves garlic
Salt and freshly ground pepper to taste
1½ to 2 tablespoons wine vinegar

1. Slip the skins off the beets and allow them to cool. Cut the beets into chunks.
2. Combine the cooled beets and all remaining ingredients in a food processor. Process until puréed (the texture will remain somewhat

rough). Taste and adjust seasonings—it should be quite peppery with a nice balance of sweet and sour. Chill.

■ *Note:* You can bake beets in the microwave (page 181).

Variation:

Stir in drained prepared horseradish and omit the garlic.

Seasoning Vegetables

Melted butter or margarine are the classic toppings for steamed vegetables. I lived for many years in the American South, where vegetables are seasoned with bacon or fatback. In the Mediterranean countries the vegetables glisten with a coating of olive oil. None of these is appropriate to the Slim Cuisine regime. What to do?

Try this. Boil *good-quality* vegetable or chicken stock until greatly reduced and syrupy, then toss with the vegetables. Even better, mix the stock with dry red or white wine, dry vermouth, or dry sherry, interesting wine vinegar, or lemon or lime juice, and then boil it down until syrupy. Add herbs or spices before you boil, but season with salt to taste *after* the boiling, or it will be much too salty.

♡ ☆ ⊕   # STEAMED BROCCOLI

Broccoli is so awful when boiled until flabby. Try it steamed briefly and rejoice in its special taste and texture.

1. Wash the head of broccoli very well. Split it into single stalks. Cut off and discard the tough ends. With a paring knife, peel the stalks up to the florets.

2. Spread the broccoli evenly in a steamer. If you love garlic, sprinkle some chopped cloves over the broccoli. Cover and steam over boiling water for 5 to 7 minutes, until crisp-tender (test with a cake tester or a toothpick). Serve at once with wedges of lemon or lime.

3. If the broccoli is to be served cold, refresh it under cold running water to stop the cooking and set the vivid green color.

Variation:

Cut the florets off the stalks. Save the stalks to serve on the next day. Steam the florets for 3 to 4 minutes over boiling water. Serve hot or cold, with lemon juice or reduced stock (see page 182).

To serve the stalks, peel them and slice ¼ inch thick and steam until tender or stir-"fry" in a small amount of stock and lemon juice until crisp-tender (see page 178 for stir-"fry" procedures).

BRAISED FENNEL

 Serves 4

Fennel looks a lot like celery and tastes like mild licorice. Braised fennel is very good as a companion to meats, or as part of a vegetable dinner.

2 fennel bulbs, trimmed and cut in half lengthwise, then each half cut into wedges about ½ inch wide	Freshly ground pepper to taste ½ cup stock 3 tablespoons grated Parmesan cheese

1. Preheat oven to 350 F.

2. Arrange the fennel in one layer (cut side down) in a baking dish. Pour ½ cup stock over it. Season with pepper. Sprinkle evenly with 3 tablespoons Parmesan cheese.

3. Bake, uncovered, for 45 minutes. The fennel will become meltingly tender and the stock will have cooked almost completely away, leaving a rich glaze. Serve at once.

♡ ☆   Omit cheese.

CHINESE BRAISED MUSHROOMS

Makes about 7 cups

Serve as a vegetable accompaniment or a starter. It works well on a buffet at a cocktail party. Because the soy sauce is salty, you won't want to add any salt as you cook the mushrooms.

3 pounds button mushrooms, cleaned
2 cups salt-free vegetable or chicken stock
½ cup dry sherry
4 tablespoons low-sodium soy sauce

1 tablespoon sugar
2 large cloves garlic, peeled and crushed
2 thin slices fresh ginger, peeled and chopped

1. Place the mushrooms in a deep heavy nonreactive pot. Add all remaining ingredients.

2. Bring to a boil. Reduce heat to a brisk simmer and cook, uncovered, stirring occasionally, until the mushrooms are deep mahogany-brown and the liquid is greatly reduced.

3. With a slotted spoon, remove the mushrooms to a bowl. Boil the remaining liquid until reduced by half. Pour the reduced liquid over the mushrooms. Serve hot or at room temperature. If they are to be part of a buffet, have cocktail picks nearby for spearing.

MUSHROOM RAGOÛT

♡ ⏱ ❄   *Makes 2¾ cups*

Serve this mushroom lover's special as a vegetable side dish or as a starter. The more kinds of mushrooms you can find, the nicer this will be.

A variety of fresh mushrooms
Freshly ground pepper to taste
Dash low-sodium soy sauce
1 to 2 tablespoons dry sherry or
  dry vermouth

½ cup stock
Purée from Baked Garlic (page 25) to taste

1. Clean mushrooms well, cut into quarters or eighths (depending on size), and combine with the remaining ingredients except the garlic purée in a large, nonstick frying pan.
2. Cook briskly until the liquid in the pan is greatly reduced.
3. Stir in the garlic purée. Cook, stirring, for a minute or so more, until the mushrooms are tender, and the sauce is syrupy. Taste and correct seasonings.

Note: Look for fresh shiitake, chestnut, and oyster mushrooms, in addition to the ordinary cultivated ones; trim the tough stems from shiitakes before using them.

♡ # BAKED POTATOES

Baked potatoes are filling, sustaining, and deeply satisfying. I've always thought that they were much too good to be relegated to the status of a mere accompaniment. For a fun, informal, and easy dinner, try serving a big napkin-lined basket of baked potatoes surrounded by an array of bowls containing all those things that go so delectably well in the potatoes. Remember, the potatoes themselves are low-fat, low-Calorie, and high in nutrition. When stuffing the potatoes, beware of wicked things like butter, sour cream, and high-fat cheeses. Instead, try a dollop of yogurt or fromage blanc, a splash of buttermilk, a billow of smoothed-out, drained cottage cheese, a modest shower of freshly grated Parmesan cheese, a squeeze of lemon juice, a scattering of herbs, a mound of Duxelles (page 187), a deluge of homemade Salsa (page 188), or a dab or so of Dijon mustard. Whatever you do, don't neglect to eat the skin. It is chock-full of nutrients, and the contrast of crunchy skin against tender flesh is part of what makes a baked potato so special.

| Large unblemished baking potatoes | Salt and freshly ground pepper to taste |

1. Preheat the oven to 425 F.

2. Scrub the potatoes and pierce them in several places with a thin skewer or the prongs of a fork. Never wrap the potatoes in foil, or they will steam rather than bake.

3. Bake directly on the oven rack for about 1¼ hours, or until the potatoes yield softly to a gentle squeeze. (Arm yourself with an oven mitt before you squeeze!)

4. Split the potatoes by perforating them lengthwise and breadthwise with the prongs of a fork and squeezing so that the tender potato flesh comes surging up. Sprinkle on a tiny bit of salt and a generous grinding of fresh black pepper and you have one of the earth's great foods at its simplest. Or serve the potatoes with the accompaniments suggested above.

Note: Baked potatoes make the most wonderful mashed potatoes. Scoop out the potato flesh (and save the skins for a private nibble). Put the potatoes through a ricer, or, for a homier (and much easier) effect, mash with a potato masher. With a wooden spoon, beat some buttermilk into the hot potatoes. Season with a touch of salt and plenty of freshly ground pepper.

DUXELLES

Makes about 2 cups

Duxelles is a kind of mushroom hash, with a very intense mushroom taste. It is useful in all sorts of preparations, so it pays to make it in quantity and store it in the refrigerator or freezer. At its most basic, try it spread thickly on bread, or stirred into sauces or soups. Better still, try it in Baked Potatoes (preceding recipe) or in ravioli (page 58). For the most intense mushroom flavor use a combination of different types of fresh mushrooms. I use shiitakes, trimmed of their tough stems, chestnut mushrooms, oyster mushrooms, and the usual cultivated ones.

2 pounds mixed mushrooms, well
   cleaned
1 cup vegetable stock
½ cup sherry
Several dashes low-sodium soy
   sauce

1 teaspoon dried tarragon,
   crumbled
Salt and freshly ground pepper to
   taste

1. Chop the mushrooms very, very fine. This is best done in a food processor if you have one. To do this, quarter the mushrooms and put them into the food processor bowl. Pulse on and off until very finely chopped. You will need to do this in 2 or more batches.

2. Empty all the chopped mushrooms into a deep, nonreactive frying pan. Add the stock, sherry, soy sauce, and tarragon. Stir it all up. The mushrooms will be barely moistened but it doesn't matter.

3. Cook over moderate heat, stirring occasionally, until the mushrooms have rendered quite a bit of liquid. Raise the heat a bit and simmer briskly, stirring occasionally, until the mushrooms are very dark, very thick, and quite dry. Season to taste. Store in the refrigerator until needed.

SALSA FOR BAKED POTATOES

♡ ☆ ◷   *Makes 2 cups*

This cold Mexican sauce spooned into steaming hot baked potatoes is very good, indeed. I also like to toss the cold salsa with hot pasta. It makes a ravishing "hot as summer, cold as winter" effect.

Two 1-pound-12-ounce cans Italian tomatoes, or 3 cups peeled and seeded fresh tomatoes in season
Finely chopped fresh chili peppers or chopped canned chiles or a mixture, to taste

¼ cup red wine vinegar
2 cloves garlic, minced
2 tablespoons chopped fresh parsley
1 tablespoon chopped fresh coriander

1. Drain the tomatoes and chop them (save the juice for soups).
2. Combine all ingredients in a nonreactive bowl. Chill.

Note: To turn this into a cold soup, use the tomato liquid as well. If you wish, add chopped roasted peppers, freshly made (page 27), or jarred.

DUXELLES CREAM FOR BAKED POTATOES

♡   *Makes 2 cups*

1 recipe Duxelles (page 187)
8 ounces quark or "smoothed-out" drained low-fat cottage cheese

2 to 3 tablespoons buttermilk

Stir the Duxelles into the quark or cottage cheese. Beat in the buttermilk.

MUSTARD CREAM FOR BAKED POTATOES

Makes ½ cup

2 tablespoons buttermilk
½ cup yogurt "Cream Cheese"
   (page 21)
2 tablespoons Dijon mustard

1 tablespoon chopped fresh
   parsley
1 tablespoon chopped fresh
   chives

Combine all the ingredients in a food processor and process until perfectly smooth. If you don't have a processor, beat the ingredients together with a wooden spoon.

BORSCHT POTATOES

One of the classic ways to serve borscht (Russian beet soup) is cold, with a steaming-hot potato in it. The hot/cold contrast is marvelous. I have reversed the classic.

Large baked potatoes
Beet Purée (page 181)

Dill sprigs for garnish (optional)

1. With a fork, perforate the hot potatoes lengthwise and breadthwise and squeeze open.
2. Pile a generous dollop of cold Beet Purée on each potato. Top each with a dill sprig. Serve at once.

STUFFED POTATOES

Serves 2 to 4

Serve these as a main course with Chinese Braised Mushrooms (page 184) and Chinese-Style Cabbage Salad (page 209) or Tomato-Basil Salad (page 204) or serve as an accompaniment to Peppered Steak (page 120). Serve 2 to 3 halves per person as a main course, 1 to 2 as an accompaniment.

1 large head garlic
2 large baking potatoes
4 ounces quark or "smoothed-out" drained cottage cheese
About 6 ounces buttermilk

4 tablespoons grated Parmesan cheese
Salt and freshly ground pepper to taste
Cayenne pepper to taste

1. Preheat the oven to 400 F.
2. Prepare the garlic heads for baking (page 23). Place the foil-wrapped garlic in the oven. Bake for 45 minutes to 1 hour.
3. Pierce potatoes in several places with a skewer or fork. Let them bake directly on the oven rack for 1 to 1¼ hours, while the garlic bakes.
4. Meanwhile, beat together the remaining ingredients. When the garlic is done, squeeze the softened pulp into the cheese mixture.
5. When the potatoes are done, cut them in half lengthwise. Scoop the potato flesh into a bowl. Be very careful to leave the potato shells intact. Mash the potatoes with a masher. With a wooden spoon, beat in the cheese-garlic mixture. Beat in more buttermilk, if necessary, to make a very creamy mixture. Taste and adjust seasonings.
6. Pile the potato mixture into the potato shells. Place them in a baking dish. (The recipe may be prepared up to this point and refrigerated. Return to room temperature before continuing.)
7. Place the baking dish in the hot oven. Bake for 10 to 15 minutes. If the potato mixture has not browned lightly on the top at this point, put it briefly under the broiler. Serve at once.

♡   Omit Parmesan cheese.

POTATO CASES

♡ ☆

Potato Cases are perfect if you crave fries or chips. They are crunchy and just right for potato-snack needs. If you wish, cut them in quarters instead of halves. They will bake faster and be more like finger food.

Large baking potatoes

1. Preheat the oven to 400 F.
2. Scrub the potatoes and halve them lengthwise.
3. With a teaspoon or a melon-baller, scoop out the insides, leaving a shell about ¼ inch thick. Save the scraps for another use (see recipe below).
4. Bake directly on the oven rack for 25 to 35 minutes, until golden brown and very crisp. Serve at once—as they are; with dips; or filled with a savory mixture.

Note: Don't you dare throw the potato scraps away. Use them to make a wonderful gratin. It may be made at once, refrigerated, and reheated at a later date.

POTATO SCRAP GRATIN

1. Scoop the potatoes right into a saucepan and add enough stock to barely cover. Season with a bit of salt and plenty of pepper. If you wish, you may add a bit of grated nutmeg or a pinch of ground cumin and cayenne pepper. Simmer, covered, until tender. Do not drain.
2. Mash roughly (just to chop up the pieces, not to purée them) right in the pot with a potato masher. Spread the mixture into a gratin dish. Dribble on a bit of skim milk, and sprinkle with some Parmesan. Bake, in a hot oven, uncovered, for 50 minutes to 1 hour, until bubbly and well browned on top. Serve at once, or refrigerate for reheating in 1 to 2 days.

POTATO GRATIN

Serves 6 to 8

This gratin is a symphony of texture and taste. The starch in the potatoes, the flavorful stock, and the grated cheese form a thick, creamy sauce that binds the tender potato slices under a crusty top.

1 large clove garlic
4 large baking potatoes, unpeeled
4 tablespoons freshly grated
  Parmesan cheese

Salt and freshly ground pepper to
  taste
1½ cups salt-free vegetable or
  chicken stock

1. Preheat the oven to 400 F.
2. Peel the garlic clove and split it. Rub a 9-x-13-inch oval gratin dish with the split sides of the garlic.
3. Slice the potatoes paper-thin. Do not soak them in water at any time. Slice just before using.
4. Layer one-third of the potato slices in the gratin dish and sprinkle evenly with Parmesan cheese, salt, and pepper. Pour one-third of the stock over the potatoes.
5. Repeat twice more. With a broad spatula, press the top layer down into the liquid.
6. Bake in the preheated oven for approximately 1½ hours, until the potatoes are tender, the liquid has cooked down to a thick sauce, and the top is brown and crusty.

♡ Omit cheese.

Note: The gratin can be made the morning or the day before and reheated in a microwave or a 375 F oven.

Variations:

1. Layer Browned Onions (page 16) with the potatoes, cheese, and stock. Cook as directed.
2. Mix 1 tablespoon Dijon mustard with ½ cup whiskey. Stir in the stock. Proceed and bake as directed.

3. Layer Sautéed Mushrooms (page 20) with the potatoes. For pure luxury, add soaked, drained, dried mushrooms, and use some of the strained mushroom liquor for part of the stock.

GRATIN OF BAKED POTATOES, ONIONS, AND GARLIC

Makes 4 cups

I invented this dish for a book I wrote a few years ago, *Comfort Food*. I have cut out the high-fat ingredients of the original recipe, but it is still one of the most comforting recipes I know.

4 large baking potatoes, baked
 and mashed (save skins for
 another use)
Purée from 2 large heads of
 baked garlic (see page 25)
2 large Spanish onions, baked and
 puréed (page 26)
Salt and freshly ground pepper to
 taste

2 to 3 tablespoons buttermilk
4 to 5 tablespoons freshly grated
 Parmesan cheese
1 tablespoon instant dried skim
 milk powder
3 tablespoons stock

1. Preheat the oven to 325 F.

2. Combine the potato, garlic, onions, salt, and pepper. Beat with a wooden spoon. Beat in the buttermilk.

3. Scrape the mixture into a gratin dish. Smooth the top and sprinkle with the cheese. (The recipe may be prepared in advance to this stage and refrigerated, covered, for a few days. Bring to room temperature before proceeding.) Whisk together the milk powder and the stock. Dribble the mixture evenly over the top of the potatoes. Bake, uncovered, for 35 to 45 minutes, until brown, bubbly, and thoroughly hot. Serve at once. (This is very exciting when it is cold, too.)

♡   Omit cheese.

FRENCH-"FRIED" POTATOES

173 Calories for fries from one
8-ounce potato
0.2g fat
(Traditional fries: 270 Calories per 8-
ounce potato, 13g fat)

Why deprive yourself of chips or fries? You can feast on these compelling munchies to your heart's content, if you use no fat. They are actually superior to the usual fat-laden kind because, as you munch, you taste *potato*, not a mouthful of grease and salt. The potatoes may be sliced thick (½ inch) or thin (¼ inch). The thin ones will be crisp and crunchy like chips, the thicker ones will be brown and crunchy on the outside and floury-tender within, like fries.

Baking potatoes	**Low-fat vegetable spray or**
Warm stock	**nonstick cooking spray**

1. Preheat the oven to 425 F.
2. Don't bother to peel the potatoes. Cut them crosswise into ¼- to ½-inch slices. Cut each slice in half.
3. Put a little bit of warm stock in a large bowl along with the potatoes and stir them around well with your hands so that they are coated with the warm stock.
4. You will need 1 or 2 flat nonstick baking sheets. Spray them with nonstick cooking spray. Spread the potatoes on the sheet(s) in one layer. Put them in the oven and leave them for 30 minutes. (Shake the pan occasionally to keep them from sticking.)
5. Pull the potatoes out and, with a spatula, gently turn them. Bake in the oven for approximately another 5 to 15 minutes. (The timing depends on the thickness of the slices.) By this time they should be browned, crunchy, and puffed. Serve at once. (These may be sprinkled with a bit of salt, if desired, but I find they don't really need it.)

ROAST POTATOES WITH ROASTED GARLIC AND ONION

♡

Serves 4

Melting tenderness and superb flavor with no fat at all. As they bake, the kitchen is filled with the most tantalizing aroma.

1 head fresh, firm garlic
3 medium onions, halved and
   sliced into thin half-moons
8 medium new potatoes,
   unpeeled and cut in half

About ¾ cup stock
Salt and freshly ground pepper to
   taste

1. Preheat oven to 400 F.
2. Separate the head of garlic into cloves. Hit each clove sharply with a kitchen mallet. Remove and discard the skin. Scatter the crushed cloves and the onion slices on the bottom of a baking dish that will hold the potatoes in one layer.
3. Place the potatoes, cut sides down, on the bed of garlic and onions. Pour in stock to come about one-quarter up the sides of the dish. Sprinkle salt and pepper evenly over all.
4. Bake, uncovered, for 1 hour, until the potatoes are tender, the onions are beginning to brown, and the liquid is about gone. Serve piping hot. Encourage diners to mash the garlic, onion, and potatoes together, if they wish.

CURRIED ROAST POTATOES

♡

Serves 4 as an accompaniment;
2 as a main dish

With plenty of Cucumber Raita (page 203) these would make a good meal. No meat is needed.

1 large onion, cut in half and each half cut into eighths
About 2 cups stock
1 thin slice fresh ginger, minced
1 teaspoon ground coriander
1 teaspoon ground cumin
½ teaspoon cayenne pepper
1 clove garlic, crushed
Salt and pepper to taste
4 medium potatoes, unpeeled and quartered
Wedges of fresh lime

1. Preheat oven to 400 F. Separate the segments of the onion pieces and spread them in a heavy frying pan. Add *no* liquid or fat. Heat the frying pan gently. Cook at moderate heat, without stirring, for 7 to 10 minutes, until the onions are sizzling, speckled with dark amber, and beginning to stick to the pan.

2. Stir in 1¼ cups stock and let it bubble up, stirring up the browned bits in the pan with a wooden spoon as it bubbles. Stir in the ginger, spices, and garlic. Reduce the heat a bit and simmer, stirring frequently, until the mixture is very thick (not at all soupy) and the onions and spices are "frying" in their own juices. Don't rush this step; it is essential that the spices should not have a raw, harsh taste. Taste and cook very gently for a few more minutes, if necessary.

3. Toss the potatoes into the mixture and stir to combine everything very well. Scrape the potatoes and spices into a shallow baking dish that can hold them in one layer. Add the remaining stock.

4. Bake at 400 F for 1 hour, stirring occasionally and adding a bit more stock as needed, until the potatoes are tender. The finished dish should be dry. Serve hot with wedges of lime.

MASHED POTATOES

Nothing helps you drift into serene calm faster than a steaming bowl-ful of this magical food. Conventionally prepared, the mashed spuds are usually loaded with cream and butter, producing sensual pleasure as you eat, followed by guilt and fat the next day. Let's keep the sensual pleasure and eliminate the guilt and fat.

To make perfect mashed potatoes, choose large baking potatoes. They have a floury texture when cooked, and mash up into a fluffy, ethereal cloud. Avoid waxy boiling potatoes; they become a sticky mass when mashed. Boil the baking potatoes in plenty of salted water in a covered pot until very tender but *not* falling apart. You will obtain the best results as far as taste and nutrition are concerned if the potatoes are boiled whole and unpeeled; but, if you are in a hurry, they may be peeled and quartered before boiling.

When the potatoes are tender, drain them in a colander. (If you love to bake bread, save the potato liquid. It is excellent for bread dough.) If the potatoes are whole and unpeeled, grasp them with an oven mitt and scrape off the skins with a table knife. Quarter them and return to the pot. If they were already peeled and quartered, simply return them to the pot directly after draining.

Cover the pot and shake it over low heat to toss the potatoes as they dry. For exceptionally fluffy, airy mashed potatoes, force them through a ricer into a warm bowl. For homier, denser potatoes, use a potato masher, and mash them right in the pan over very low heat. Work the potatoes well with the masher. It is all right to leave in a lump or two, to prove that these are *real* mashed potatoes, but watch out for rampant lumpiness or they will be awful. Don't be tempted to use your food processor; you'll end up with a gluey mess.

When the potatoes are mashed or riced, season to taste with salt and pepper. (For a really interesting, if unconventional, taste, add a bit of ground cumin and cayenne pepper, too.) With a wooden spoon, beat in a liberal amount of room-temperature buttermilk until they look creamy and luxurious. A bit of freshly grated Parmesan cheese can be beaten in too, if you wish.

♡   Omit the Parmesan cheese.

Variations:

1. Add one of the following vegetables to mashed potatoes (steam or bake the vegetables and use an equal weight of the vegetable and of potatoes): mashed rutabagas; mashed parsnips; mashed turnips; mashed carrots; mashed celeriac.

2. Or stir in: Browned Onions (page 16); Puréed Baked Onion (page 26); Baked Garlic Purée (page 25); chopped chives

3. Or, for a delectable potato experience, fill a bowl with mashed potatoes. Make a well in the potatoes with the back of a spoon. Fill the well with Sautéed Mushrooms (page 20) or Mushroom Ragoût (page 185).

4. Or make a Mashed Potato Gratin: Mash the potatoes, beat in plenty of buttermilk and a bit of Parmesan, season with salt, freshly ground black pepper, a sprinkle of cayenne pepper, and a couple of pinches of ground cumin. Spread the mixture in a gratin dish. Dribble a bit of skim milk evenly over the surface and sprinkle with some grated Parmesan. (It may be made in advance to this point and refrigerated. Bring to room temperature before proceeding.) Bake at 400 F for 45 minutes to 1 hour, until puffed with a golden crust.

SPICY LENTILS

Makes 7 cups

This makes a *lot* of lentils, but it freezes or refrigerates well and tastes so good upon reheating. If you wish, dilute the leftovers with plenty of stock to make a delicious soup.

2 large onions, cut into eighths
About 6 cups stock
1 tablespoon minced fresh ginger
1 clove garlic, minced
1 teaspoon ground cinnamon
1 teaspoon ground coriander
Cayenne pepper to taste

1 pound brown lentils, washed
   and picked over
2 large limes
Salt to taste
Chopped fresh coriander for
   garnish (optional)

1. Separate the segments of the onion pieces and spread them in a heavy, nonstick frying pan. Add *no* liquid or fat. Heat the frying pan gently. Cook at moderate heat, without stirring, for 7 to 10 minutes, until the onions are sizzling, speckled with dark amber, and beginning to stick to the pan.

2. Stir in 1¼ cups stock and let it bubble up, stirring up the browned bits in the pan with a wooden spoon as it bubbles. Stir in the ginger, garlic, and spices. Reduce the heat a bit and simmer, stirring frequently, until the mixture is very thick (not at all soupy), and the onions and spices are "frying" in their own juices. Don't rush this step; it is essential that the spices should not have a raw, harsh taste. Taste and cook very gently for a few more minutes, if necessary.

3. Add the lentils. Stir so that they are coated with the onions and spices. Cut the limes in half and squeeze the juice into the lentils. Add the squeezed halves to the pan. (Discard before serving.) Pour in 4 cups stock.

4. Simmer, uncovered, for 10 minutes. Skim off the foam as it comes to the surface.

5. Cover and simmer gently, stirring occasionally, for 45 to 50 minutes. Add more stock during this time, as needed, and salt halfway through.

6. Taste the lentils. If they are not quite tender, add more stock and simmer for 15 to 20 minutes, until completely tender and the mixture is hot. Taste and add more salt and lime juice, if necessary. Serve hot, garnished with chopped coriander, if desired.

SALADS AND DRESSINGS

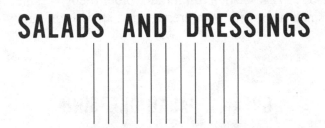

Salads often seduce dieters into outrageous overindulgence. Although everyone knows that salads are perfect for chronic Calorie counters, it is easy to forget that thick, oily dressings, fried croutons, and the like are the antithesis of diet food. Leave off the densely calorific components, and salads can be a dieter's salvation. And by replacing the sludgy, oil-laden dressings with delicate, low-fat ones, the salads will be aesthetically much more pleasing.

General Guidelines for Salad Dressings

Use the Slim Cuisine "Mayonnaise" or drain low-fat fromage blanc or yogurt for an hour in a cheesecloth-lined sieve. Mix it with a splash of freshly squeezed lemon or orange juice or wine vinegar.

To this basic mixture may be added minced raw garlic or roasted garlic purée, chopped fresh herbs, ground spices, grated citrus zest, grated fresh ginger, minced shallots or scallions, a dash of low-sodium soy sauce or Worcestershire (look for reduced-salt Worcestershire in health-food shops), Dijon mustard, a few dashes of Tabasco sauce, minced capers, a dab of tomato paste (for a "Russian" dressing), or prepared horseradish. Choose the flavoring to complement the salad.

For a creamy, zesty dressing, try mixing 2 to 3 parts of drained low-fat yogurt to one part Dijon mustard with a splash or two of interesting vinegar (balsamic, raspberry, sherry, herb, et cetera). In fact, the more interesting vinegars, particularly sherry and balsamic, make good dressings all by themselves.

If you love to eat salad in restaurants, order them without dressings. Carry a small jar of your own dressing and apply it discreetly.

 ## CREAMY SALAD DRESSING

Salads are full of fiber, low-fat, low-Calorie, vitamin- and mineral-packed veggies, and, alas, usually drenched in horrifically high-fat dressings. How nice to know that you can have your creamy salad dressing minus the fat by using Slim Cuisine "Mayonnaise" as a base.

Wine vinegar (see note)
Buttermilk

"Mayonnaise" (page 22)

Whisk the vinegar and a bit of buttermilk into the "Mayonnaise" in a thin stream until the consistency of light cream.

Vary this dressing to your taste with garlic, herbs, spices, et cetera. A specific example follows.

Note: Use as interesting a vinegar as you can find and afford. Sherry, balsamic, or raspberry vinegars are excellent. White wine tarragon vinegar works nicely too.

CREAMY HERB SALAD DRESSING

Makes 1 cup

Try this variation of the preceding recipe on a special tossed salad—for instance, green and red lettuces tossed with chicory leaves, strips of red and yellow bell peppers, watercress, and orange segments.

½ cup yogurt "Cream Cheese" (page 21)
4 tablespoons buttermilk
1 to 2 tablespoons Dijon mustard
1½ tablespoons sherry vinegar
2 cloves crushed garlic (optional)
2 tablespoons fresh basil leaves
Salt and freshly ground pepper to taste

Combine all the ingredients in the container of a food processor. Process until smooth. Scrape into a jar, cover tightly, and refrigerate until needed.

CUCUMBER RAITA

Makes about 2½ cups

Always serve a cooling raita (yogurt salad) with your curries. Here are my favorites.

2½ cups low-fat yogurt
1 large cucumber, peeled, halved, and seeded
Salt and freshly ground pepper to taste
Chopped fresh parsley
Chopped fresh coriander
Thinly sliced scallions (green and white portions)
Chili powder (optional)

1. Place yogurt in a bowl.
2. Grate the cucumber into the yogurt.
3. Stir to combine. Season to taste with salt and pepper. Garnish generously with chopped parsley, chopped coriander, and sliced scallions. Sprinkle on chili powder, if desired. Serve at once as an accompaniment to curries.

Variation: MINT RAITA

♡ ◔ Mix plenty of chopped fresh mint with yogurt. Omit the cucumbers and the coriander.

♡ ORANGE-WATERCRESS SALAD

This is a beautiful and refreshing salad, perfect for warm weather. Plan on ½ orange per person, a few sprigs of watercress, and a teaspoon of dressing. For a stunning presentation, arrange the salad on clear glass plates.

Juicy seedless oranges
Watercress, washed and shaken
  dry
Low-fat yogurt, drained for about
  1 hour

Freshly ground pepper
½ teaspoon grated orange rind
Pinch ground cumin

1. On a cutting board, thinly slice the oranges. With a paring knife, neatly remove the rind and white pith from each slice. Do not wipe away the orange juice that collects on the board.

2. Overlap the orange slices on half of a clear glass plate. Fan out the watercress on the lower half. Stir the orange juice that has collected on the cutting board into the drained yogurt along with the pepper, orange rind, and cumin. Either serve the dressing in a clear glass pitcher along with the salad, or pour a thin stripe of dressing down the center of each row of orange slices, and serve the rest separately.

♡ ☆ ◷ TOMATO-BASIL SALAD

Tomato and basil form a heavenly culinary alliance. Make the most of this duo during the summer, when both are in glorious profusion. For a more substantial salad, alternate slices of tomato with slices of part-skim mozzarella cheese.

Ripe tomatoes
Basil leaves, torn into shreds
Salt and freshly ground pepper

Sherry vinegar or other good,
  mild wine vinegar

1. Neatly cut the stem out of the tomatoes. Slice them from stem to stern. Arrange the slices on a plate. Sprinkle lightly with salt and pepper.

2. Scatter the shredded basil over the tomatoes. Sprinkle on a modest amount of vinegar. Let stand for 10 minutes before serving.

MARINATED CUCUMBER SALAD

Makes 2 cups

This is a low-fat version of a classic Hungarian salad. The creamy variation is especially good with broiled flank steak or roasted chicken. Serve it on the same plate as the meat, so that the meat juices mingle with the salad.

2 large cucumbers, peeled
Salt
3 tablespoons white wine vinegar
½ teaspoon sugar
½ teaspoon Hungarian paprika or
   paprika paste

Freshly ground pepper to taste
1 small clove garlic, crushed
   (optional)

1. Thinly slice the cucumber into a colander. Toss lightly with salt and let drain for approximately 30 minutes. Rinse and blot dry on paper towels.

2. Meanwhile, whisk together the vinegar, 3 tablespoons water, the sugar, ¼ teaspoon paprika, the pepper, and garlic. Mix this dressing into the rinsed, drained cucumbers. Chill for 1 hour or so before serving. Just before serving, sprinkle the remaining paprika over the top of the salad.

Creamy Variation:

Stir in some yogurt or fromage blanc until it is as creamy as you like.

LUXURIOUS POTATO SALAD

♡ ◷

Makes 5 cups

What an elegant and delicious combination: the warm potatoes soak up the ambrosial balsamic vinegar; the stock becomes imbued with the intense taste of the sun-dried tomatoes; the chili peppers provide a slight bite; the turkey imparts a subtle smokiness. All in all, a potato salad to cherish. Who needs mayonnaise? The mere thought is ludicrous!

1½ pounds small new potatoes, halved or quartered, depending on size
1 large clove garlic, halved
3 ounces smoked turkey breast, finely diced
1 tablespoon drained capers
1 grilled pepper (page 27), diced, or jarred pepper
2 tablespoons balsamic vinegar
1¼ cups chicken stock
3 to 4 dry-pack sun-dried

tomatoes, finely snipped (use scissors)
1 or 2 pinches dried red pepper flakes
Freshly ground black pepper to taste
2 tablespoons chopped fresh parsley
3 scallions, trimmed, cut in half lengthwise, then thinly sliced crosswise

1. Steam the potatoes until tender but not falling apart.
2. Rub a glass or ceramic bowl thoroughly with the cut sides of the garlic. Discard the garlic.
3. Toss the potatoes, smoked turkey, capers, and pepper in the bowl. Toss in the balsamic vinegar.
4. Combine the stock, sun-dried tomatoes, and pepper flakes in a small frying pan. Boil rapidly until reduced by half.
5. Immediately pour the reduced stock mixture over the potatoes. With a wooden spoon, turn the potatoes so that they are coated with the stock mixture. Season with black pepper, and toss in the parsley and scallions. Serve at once, or store in the refrigerator until needed.

CHICK-PEA–POTATO SALAD

Makes 4 cups

This is a lively potato salad. It would be excellent as part of a vegetarian meal.

1 pound boiling potatoes
One 15-ounce can chick-peas
2 tablespoons fresh lime juice
1 teaspoon low-sodium soy sauce
½ teaspoon ground cumin
¼ teaspoon cayenne pepper, or less if you don't like things spicy

3 scallions, trimmed and thinly sliced
2 tablespoons chopped fresh parsley
3 tablespoons drained yogurt or fromage blanc
1 tablespoon buttermilk

1. Steam the potatoes until tender but not mushy. Cut into ½-inch cubes while still warm.

2. Rinse and drain the chick-peas. Combine them in a bowl with the potatoes. Stir together the lime juice, soy sauce, and spices. Add this mixture to the potatoes and toss gently with 2 spoons, so that they absorb the liquid. Stir in the scallions and parsley.

3. Stir together the yogurt and buttermilk, then gently fold the mixture into the potatoes. Serve at once, or store in the refrigerator until needed.

FENNEL-PEPPER SALAD

Serves 4

The licorice crunchiness of fennel makes this salad exceptionally pleasing. Serve it as a separate course, either before or after the main dish.

1 medium head fennel, trimmed
of tough outer layer and core,
and sliced thin (save feathery
leaves)
1 small red bell pepper, peeled
(page 179) and sliced thin
1 small yellow bell pepper,
peeled and sliced thin
¼ pound button mushrooms,
cleaned well and sliced thin

1 tablespoon capers, rinsed and
drained
2 large cloves garlic
½ cup chopped fresh parsley
¼ cup "Mayonnaise" (page 22)
1 to 2 tablespoons buttermilk
1 tablespoon wine vinegar

1. Combine the fennel, peppers, mushrooms, and capers in a bowl.

2. Finely chop together the garlic and parsley. Toss them, along with the feathery fennel leaves, into the vegetables.

3. Whisk together the "Mayonnaise," buttermilk, and vinegar. Toss the dressing with the salad, or pass it in a clear glass pitcher. Serve at once.

CORN SALAD

Makes 8 cups

Corn Salad will keep in the refrigerator for several days, and improve in flavor day by day. I make this with thawed frozen corn. The recipe is at its best prepared with grilled fresh peppers, but jarred red peppers will do when time is short. In fact, you could use canned tomatoes, too, but the salad is so much more scintillating with fresh, ripe beauties.

1 pound frozen kernel sweet
corn, thawed and microwaved
or steamed until just tender
6 fresh ripe tomatoes, peeled,
seeded, juiced, and coarsely
chopped

6 grilled, peeled red bell peppers
(see page 179), coarsely
chopped (or use jarred red
peppers)
¼ cup diced canned hot chiles, or
1 to 2 fresh chiles, chopped

Salt and freshly ground pepper to
taste
2 tablespoons balsamic or wine
vinegar

2 tablespoons each: chopped
fresh coriander and chopped
fresh parsley

Combine all ingredients in a shallow dish, tossing them together.
Chill, stirring occasionally. Serve cold.

CHINESE-STYLE CABBAGE SALAD

Makes 3½ cups

This is an approximation of the cabbage salad my friend Frank Ma
used to serve me at his Chinese restaurant in Atlanta, Georgia. I have
adapted it somewhat, but the salad still has the authentic Chinese
taste.

¾ pound green cabbage, shredded
2 large carrots, shredded
4 tablespoons fresh lime or lemon
juice
1 teaspoon sugar

1 small clove garlic, crushed
Cayenne pepper to taste
1 tablespoon low-sodium soy
sauce

1. Combine cabbage and carrots in a large bowl.
2. Whisk together the remaining ingredients. Add the dressing to
the vegetables and toss with 2 spoons, so that the cabbage is well-
coated with the dressing. Let stand for at least 15 minutes before serving, stirring occasionally.

TABOULI

Makes 6 cups

Tabouli is a salad of herbs, tomatoes, and grain. The colorful mixture is extraordinarily refreshing. The success of the dish depends on the tomatoes; they must be ripe and bursting with flavor. Tabouli goes very well with broiled fish, chicken, or meat, or with lamb meatballs. And it makes a pretty addition to a salad buffet. Bulghur is available in most health-food stores.

1½ cups cracked wheat (bulghur)
½ cup fresh lemon juice
2 cups stemmed and finely chopped fresh parsley
1 bunch scallions, trimmed and finely chopped
½ cup finely shredded fresh mint
2 pounds ripe tomatoes, skinned (see page 42), seeded, juiced, and chopped
Salt and freshly ground pepper to taste

1. Soak the bulghur in cold water to cover. Use a large bowl, because it will expand a great deal. After 30 minutes, squeeze the grains with your hands to drain and place them in a clean bowl.
2. Stir in the lemon juice, and all remaining ingredients. Mix well. Let sit for at least 1 hour before serving.

ONION-TOMATO RELISH

Makes about 2 cups

A vibrant sweet and sour relish that is a perfect addition to barbecues and picnics. It's the 20 cloves of gently cooked garlic that give it such pizzazz.

4 ounces raisins
½ cup dark rum
20 large cloves garlic, peeled and sliced
About ¾ cup stock
1½ pounds frozen pearl onions, unthawed

¾ cup apple juice	Salt and freshly ground pepper to
1-pound can chopped Italian	taste
tomatoes	

1. Combine the raisins and rum in a small bowl, and set aside.

2. Combine the garlic and ½ cup stock in a large heavy nonreactive frying pan. Boil, uncovered, until the stock is thick and syrupy and the garlic is very tender.

3. Add the frozen onions and 3 fluid ounces apple juice. Simmer briskly, uncovered, until the mixture is almost dry and the onions are beginning to brown. Add the remaining apple juice and continue cooking, shaking the pan occasionally until the onions are browned and glazed.

4. Add a splash of stock. Simmer, shaking the frying pan for a few minutes, until the onions are deeply and evenly browned.

5. Stir in the tomatoes, salt, and pepper. Stir in the raisins and the rum. Simmer gently, covered, for 40 minutes, until the mixture is very thick and the onions are very tender. Uncover to stir occasionally. Add a bit of stock if the mixture gets thick too early and threatens to burn.

6. Store in the refrigerator. Bring to room temperature before serving.

EGGPLANT RELISH

 Makes about 2 cups

This is a variant of "poor man's caviar," a rich eggplant spread that appears in many guises in the cuisines of the Middle East and Eastern Europe. Usually such concoctions contain oceans of oil—here baking the garlic, the eggplant, and grilling the peppers give vivid flavor and unctuous texture despite the missing oil. It's great spread on pumpernickel slices.

Flesh from 2 small baked
  eggplants (page 28) (¾ pound
  each), coarsely chopped
Purée from 1 large head baked
  garlic (page 25)
2 red bell peppers, grilled, peeled,
  and chopped (page 179), or use
  jarred peppers
1 large ripe tomato, peeled,
  seeded, and chopped, or 2 or 3
  canned Italian tomatoes,
  drained and chopped

Juice of ½ lemon
2 to 4 scallions, trimmed, cut in
  half lengthwise, and sliced thin
  crosswise
8 tablespoons chopped fresh
  parsley
3 tablespoons chopped fresh mint
Salt and freshly ground pepper to
  taste
Chopped fresh parsley for garnish

1. Combine all the ingredients except garnish in the bowl of a food processor. Pulse the machine on and off, until the mixture has formed a rough purée. Taste and adjust seasonings, adding more salt, pepper, and lemon juice as needed.

2. Scrape into a glass or ceramic bowl and chill until needed. At serving time, garnish with additional chopped parsley.

SNACKS AND SANDWICHES

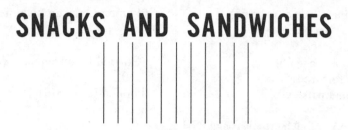

It's the cravings and snackings and in-between munchings that get you into trouble. Little crispy fried things scarfed down in frightening quantity; butter- and mayonnaise-smeared sandwiches overstuffed with fatty meats; oily, sausage-festooned pizzas; "fun" foods, but so bad for your weight maintenance and your health. Apply Slim Cuisine techniques to your snacking, and you can still have fun. After all, a sandwich is one of the friendliest edible objects in the world. There's something about two pieces of bread slapped together with interesting (and sometimes eccentric) ingredients that can cheer up the dourest snacker. Why deprive yourself? And why miss out on crispy little munchies, on pizza, on nachos? Read on.

Slim Sandwiches

For your sandwiches use a good whole-grain sliced bakery loaf that has some character, a crusty rye, or a moist black bread.

Sliced chicken (roasted, smoked, or poached)
Tomatoes

Creamy Pesto (page 160)

♡ Tzatziki (page 63)
Smoked salmon

Sliced cucumber
Dill Pesto (page 161)

| 213 |

♡ Liptauer Cheese (page 60)
Sliced turkey

♡ Tonnato sauce (page 65)
Roasted peppers

Hummus (page 66)
Sliced tomatoes
Chopped parsley

Broiled Lamb Meatballs (page 99)
   or Kofta Curry (page 103)
Cucumber or Mint Raita (page
   203)
Served in pita bread pockets:

Italian Sausage Balls (page 105)

Tomato Sauce (page 166)
Stir-"fried" or grilled peppers
Served in pita bread pockets or
   Italian bread

♡ Dill chicken salad
Sliced tomatoes

♡ Lemon Chicken (page 146)
Chive spread

♡ Curried Chicken Salad (page
   130)
Chopped fresh coriander
Sliced mango

Peppered flank steak slices
Browned Onions (page 16) or
   Sweet-and-Sour Onions (page
   19)
Mustard

♡ Pan-Sautéed Chicken Cutlet
   (page 128)
Stir-"fried" peppers

SLIM REUBEN

Sliced smoked chicken
Rinsed and drained sauerkraut
Thinly sliced part-skim
   mozzarella cheese

"Russian" dressing
   ("Mayonnaise," page 22, mixed
   with a bit of tomato paste)

Toast this sandwich in a toaster oven.

CLUB SANDWICH

♡

"Mayonnaise" (page 22)
Smoked chicken

Sliced tomato
Lettuce

Toast the bread first.

SUMMER SANDWICH

Sliced tomatoes
Quark or thinly sliced part-skim
   mozzarella cheese

Fresh basil and chopped garlic
A light sprinkling of excellent
   wine vinegar (optional)

LUXURIOUS SUMMER SANDWICH

Chop together fresh basil, fresh garlic, and Parmesan cheese, and put
this mixture on 1 slice of whole-grain bread. Top with sliced ripe
tomatoes and thin slices of mozzarella. Sprinkle on some minced sun-
dried tomatoes. Toast this sandwich in a toaster oven.

PIZZA SANDWICH

Thinly sliced part-skim mozzarella cheese
Tomato sauce
Shredded fresh or crumbled dried
   oregano
Crumbled dried chili peppers
   (optional)

A spoonful of Sautéed
   Mushrooms (page 20) (optional)
A few slices of peeled red and
   yellow bell peppers (optional)

Toast this sandwich in a toaster oven.

VEGETARIAN SANDWICH I

Beet Purée (page 181) or Baked Beets in mustard sauce (see page 180)

Watercress

VEGETARIAN SANDWICH II

Chopped raw fresh spinach
Sliced raw mushrooms

Dijon mustard mixed with yogurt

Use black bread for this sandwich.

GOOD SPREADS FOR HONEST BREAD

These are marvelous on slices of toasted whole-grain or rye bread.

Garlic spread (quark mixed with baked Garlic Purée, page 25, and a touch of finely grated Parmesan. Vary with grated nutmeg, chopped fresh herbs, or chopped chives or scallions)
Beet Purée (page 181)
Duxelles (page 187)

ELLE GALE'S SARDINE FISH CREAM

Makes 1 cup

I make this with skim goat's milk curd cheese, but it's also good with quark, "smoothed-out" drained cottage cheese, or any other low-fat curd cheese. Mash together 4 ounces low-fat curd cheese with the contents of a 4-ounce can of sardines in tomato sauce (check the label and make sure it contains no oil). Stir in 2 teaspoons chopped chives; 2 scallions, chopped; 3 dashes low-sodium Worcestershire sauce; 1 teaspoon lemon juice; salt and pepper to taste.

CHEESE ON TOAST

Lightly toast a piece of rye bread. Cut a clove of garlic in half. Rub the hot toast with the garlic halves. Cover the toast thinly with sliced part-skim mozzarella cheese. Broil for 2 to 3 minutes, until melted and speckled with brown. Sprinkle lightly with Hungarian paprika. Devour at once.

PIZZA

Pizza, with its gooey cheese and spicy sauce, may not be elegant, but it is one of the most satisfying dishes in the world. Happily, it is also one of the healthiest, if you avoid additions such as sausage, ham, and other fatty meats.

When you are eating pizza out, specify that your pizza be prepared with no oil and no salt. The pizza will still be sumptuous, yet your Slim Cuisine regime will stay intact.

It's fun to make pizza at home and easy, too, if you begin with pita bread as your base. Leave the pita as it is or, to cut the Calories even more, split each pita into 2 rounds. Place the pita on the broiler tray (if they are split, place them smooth side down). Smear with Slim Cuisine Tomato Sauce (page 166) and top with thin slices of part-skim mozzarella cheese. If possible, use the Italian-type brands that come packed in water. If you wish, top the sauce with Sautéed Mushrooms (page 20), Browned Onions (page 16), sliced Meatballs (page 104), or Stir-"Fried" Yellow and Red Peppers (page 179) before laying on the cheese. Sprinkle on a little oregano. Have the broiler set to its highest setting and place the broiler tray in the lowest position. Broil for 3 to 4 minutes, until the cheese is nicely gooey and runny. Eat with pleasure and no guilt at all.

♡ # TORTILLA CHIPS

Tortilla chips, sometimes called nacho chips (*totopos* in Mexico), are very popular as snack food. They are compelling munchies on their own, or as paddles for dips. Alas, they are always fried and often oversalted, too. Make your own healthy tortilla chips with no frying and only as much salt as you want. You can buy refrigerated, frozen, or canned tortillas. Bake as many tortillas as you like, in one layer, on the rack of your oven at 300 F for 15 to 20 minutes, until crisp. Remove them and break into eighths. (Alternately, for neater pieces, cut the tortillas in quarters or eighths with scissors *before* baking. Spread the pieces directly on the oven rack.) Sprinkle with a bit of salt, or chili powder, paprika, cumin, whatever you like. Or leave unseasoned so that the pure and heady corn taste comes through. Store in an airtight container. Eat as they are, use with dips, or consider one of the following preparations.

■ *Microwave Version:*

   1. Put a double layer of paper towels on the microwave carousel.
   2. Arrange 5 tortillas around the periphery of the towels, without letting them touch each other. Microwave at full power for 2 to 2½ minutes.
   3. If the towels are wet, replace them. Turn the tortillas over and microwave at full power for another 2 to 2½ minutes.
   4. Remove the chips to a rack and allow to rest for 5 minutes. Break into quarters or eighths, and store in an airtight container.

TOSTADAS

1. Spread *whole* baked tortillas with Chili con Carne (page 113) and sprinkle with shredded part-skim mozzarella. Broil for 1 to 2 minutes, to melt the cheese. Serve at once.

2. Spread the whole baked tortilla with mashed, cooked beans (black beans or kidney beans) that have been seasoned with salt, ground cumin, and chili powder. Sprinkle with shredded part-skim mozzarella. Broil as above. Serve at once.

3. Spread with mashed black beans or kidney beans that have been thinned with a bit of stock and gently warmed. Top with crisp, shredded lettuce, a dollop of yogurt or fromage blanc, and peeled and finely chopped red and yellow bell peppers (page 179).

NACHOS AL CARBON

Break the baked tortillas into quarters (or cut them into quarters with scissors before you bake them). Spread them out in one layer on a baking tray or ovenproof platter. Put a dollop of mashed black or kidney beans on each. Top with a slice of grilled flank steak. Top with shredded part-skim mozzarella. Broil for 1 minute to melt the cheese. Add a dab of yogurt or fromage blanc and some Salsa (page 188), if you wish. Place the tray in the middle of the table and let everyone grab and munch.

DESSERTS

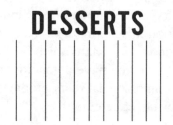

You've heard it a thousand times: desserts and sweets are evil, they will rot your teeth, pad your hips, and probably initiate moral disintegration. Don't believe it! I have a wonderful surprise for you: a whole bunch of indulgent desserts that will not contribute an iota to the decay of your teeth, or compromise your litheness or your good character. These sweets are all visual knockouts, as well as delicious. Some are "nouvelle" in character, others endearingly old-fashioned, but each will end a meal with a flourish.

Dessert Guidelines

1. Desserts should always be considered a significant and important component of a meal, not a cholesterol-, fat-, and Calorie-laden "reward" for finishing all your vegetables. Plan your desserts so that they contribute valuable nutrients along with their Calories. Worthless Calories are a Slim Cuisine no-no.

2. A little bit of sugar every once in a while will not hurt. Just remember that sugar should always be a light seasoning to be used by the sprinkle; not a major ingredient to be used by the handful. A sugar substitute can be used, preferably Aspartame, in recipes that do not call for high heat. (When heated, the sweetness in some sugar substitutes dissipates.) Whichever you choose, use it in moderation. It is a good idea to alternate sweeteners, so that you do not overload on one

or the other. If you decide to substitute sugar for Aspartame in any of these recipes, you will be adding 34 Calories per tablespoon of sugar to the Calorie count of the finished dish.

3. High-quality unsweetened frozen fruits and berries are available in exhilarating profusion in supermarkets. Keep your freezer stocked at all times with a good variety. Many splendid, nutritious desserts can be made in minutes when you have a generous supply at hand. Also keep on hand a selection of low-fat dairy products: yogurt, buttermilk, skim milk, fromage blanc, et cetera.

Ice Creams and Sorbets

Slim Cuisine ice creams are so creamy, so vividly fruity and outrageously voluptuous that you will feel delightful pangs of guilt as you polish off a large serving. Not to worry. They are nutrient-dense and Calorie-shy, so it's okay to indulge. Make them, serve them, and eat them. They do not store well. (These recipes can be halved, if desired.) Use these ideas as guidelines and invent your own versions.

BANANA ICE CREAM

                                            Serves 6

4 ripe bananas, peeled, cut into chunks, and frozen (they should be frozen so that you have separate pieces, not a large frozen mass)

½ teaspoon pure vanilla extract
Sugar substitute to taste (you will need little, if any)
½ to ¾ cup buttermilk

1. Place the frozen banana chunks in the container of a food processor. Add the vanilla, sweetener, and half the buttermilk.
2. Turn on the processor and let it run for a few moments. Then, while it is running, pour in the remaining buttermilk in a thin, steady

stream. Let the machine run until the mixture is beautifully smooth and creamy. Spoon it into bowls and serve at once.

BANANA-GINGER ICE CREAM

Follow the instructions for Banana Ice Cream (preceding recipe), but omit the vanilla extract. Add a scant teaspoon of grated fresh ginger and, if you wish, a splash of dark rum.

RASPBERRY ICE CREAM

♡ ◔   *Makes about 3 cups*

One 12-ounce package frozen unsweetened raspberries

¾ to 1 cup cold buttermilk
Sugar substitute to taste

1. Do not thaw the berries. Place them, still frozen, in the bowl of a food processor or blender. Pour in half of the buttermilk and sprinkle in a bit of sweetener.
2. Turn on the machine and process for a few seconds, stopping to scrape down the sides, if necessary. Taste for sweetness.
3. With the machine running, pour in the remaining buttermilk, and more sweetener, if necessary. Process until the mixture forms a super-creamy ice cream. Spoon into clear glass goblets and serve at once.

Variations:

1. Strawberry Ice Cream: Substitute frozen strawberries for the raspberries.

2. Strawberry-Orange Ice Cream: Add the pulp, juice, and grated zest of an orange to the berries in step 1.

3. Apple Ice Cream: Substitute frozen apple pieces and a frozen banana cut into chunks for the raspberries. Add a sprinkling of cinnamon.

♡ ⊕

PINEAPPLE SORBET

For this wonderfully refreshing recipe you need frozen pineapple cubes. Buy ripe pineapples, peel and cube them, discarding the tough core, and freeze the cubes flat on baking trays. When thoroughly frozen, transfer them to plastic bags. When you want to make sorbet, remove the amount you need. If the cubes have frozen together in the bag so that you have a solid mass, knock the bag on the counter a few times to separate them.

Frozen pineapple cubes | **1 or 2 splashes dark rum**

Place the frozen pineapple cubes and the rum in the container of a food processor. Turn the machine on. It will rattle and clatter and leap all over the counter. Steady it and allow it to run, stopping occasionally to scrape down the sides with a rubber spatula, until the pineapple cubes are of a sorbet consistency. Serve at once.

♡ ⊕

MANGO SORBET

You haven't lived until you've tasted Mango Sorbet. Use it as a stunning finish to an elegant dinner, or serve it as a private indulgence. The mango cubes can be frozen months ahead of time. (Make sure that you use really ripe mangoes.) The sorbet itself must be prepared just before serving. It's very easy and very quick. Simply excuse yourself, retire to the food processor, whip it up, and serve it forth proudly. Your guests will admire your talent and ingenuity.

Whole mangoes	a tablespoon of buttermilk, if
1 or 2 splashes dark rum	necessary
(optional)	Mint leaves for garnish
A sprinkle of sugar substitute and	

1. With a sharp knife, slice down on each whole mango as if you were slicing it in half, but try to miss the large flat center pit. Slice down again on the other side of the pit. You will now have 2 half mangoes and the flat center pit to which quite a bit of mango flesh clings.

2. With a small, sharp paring knife, score each mango half lengthwise and crosswise, cutting all the way to, but not through, the skin. Push out the skin as if you were pushing the half mango inside out. The mango flesh will stand out in cubes. Slice these cubes off the skin.

3. With the knife, remove the skin from the mango flesh remaining on the pit. Slice the flesh off the pit. Spread all the mango cubes and pieces on a flat tray and freeze. When frozen solid, transfer to plastic bags. Pull out the bags when you are ready to make the sorbet. If the cubes have frozen together in the bag, so that you have a solid mass, knock it on the counter a few times.

4. To make the sorbet, place the frozen mango cubes and the optional rum in the container of a food processor. Turn the machine on. It will rattle and clatter all over the counter. Steady it and allow it to run, stopping occasionally to scrape down the sides with a rubber spatula. The mango cubes will seem quite splintery at first. Taste for sweetness. If necessary, add a sprinkling of sugar substitute, but if the mangoes were really ripe it probably won't be necessary. Continue processing and, if the mango does not seem to be coming to sorbet consistency, add 1 to 2 tablespoons buttermilk (no more). When the mixture reaches a very smooth sorbet consistency, place several small balls of the sorbet on each plate. Garnish with mint leaves. (In the summer, a scattering of raspberries, blackberries, and other berries can be arranged on the plate as well.)

Variation:

This recipe works very well with ripe cantaloupe, too. Remove the melon flesh with a teaspoon or a melon baller and freeze the pieces flat, then transfer to plastic bags.

BLUEBERRY ICE CREAM

 Makes 3 cups

For this brilliantly colored ice cream, squirrel away blueberries in the freezer. In season, buy them in profusion, freeze them flat on trays, then transfer to plastic bags. Blueberries are usually sweet enough—but you may need the barest sprinkle of sweetener.

12 ounces frozen blueberries	Sugar substitute (optional)
¾ to 1 cup cold buttermilk	

1. Do not thaw the berries. Put them, still frozen, into the bowl of a food processor or blender. Pour in half the buttermilk.
2. Turn on the machine and process for a few seconds, stopping to scrape down the sides, if necessary. Taste. Add a bit of sweetener, if needed. Pour in the remaining buttermilk and process until the mixture forms a super-creamy ice cream. Spoon it into clear glass goblets and serve *at once*.

Note: More ice cream ideas: frozen peaches flavored with almond or vanilla extract; or try combinations: pineapple/orange, raspberry/melon, banana/strawberry.

SLIM "WHIPPED CREAM"

Makes 2¼ cups

In the summer months, seasonal fruits or berries with a creamy topping make an elegant, hard-to-improve finale to a meal. Here is the
simplest topping (and one of the best): Quickly and gently rinse some
strawberries in a colander under running water. Shake dry, and put
them, in a bowl, on the table. Give everyone a small bowl of yogurt
or fromage blanc and an even smaller bowl of dark brown sugar (1
tablespoon or less). Let everyone pick up a berry by its green top, dip
it into the yogurt or fromage blanc, then into the sugar. Eating these
delectable morsels is pure summer pleasure. If you want to get a bit
more elegant, try the following topping for fresh berries or sliced
peaches, or whatever you like—it's better than real whipped cream.
But you *must* know your eggs for this one. Because a raw egg is used
in the recipe, use only the freshest eggs, from a trusted supplier.

1 cup fromage blanc or low-fat yogurt "Cream Cheese" (page 21)	2 egg whites, at room temperature Pinch of salt
	Pinch of cream of tartar
¼ teaspoon pure vanilla extract	2 tablespoons sugar

1. Mix together the fromage blanc or yogurt and vanilla.

2. In a spotlessly clean bowl, with a wire whip, beat the egg whites
with the salt and cream of tartar until they are foamy. Add the sugar,
a little at a time, and continue beating until the egg whites are shiny
and hold firm peaks.

3. Fold the beaten egg whites into the fromage blanc or yogurt.
Serve at once.

BLACKBERRY GRATIN

Serves 8

This old-fashioned fruit *brulée* is one of my all-time favorites. Because it uses frozen berries, it can be enjoyed all the year round. A summertime recipe for fruit gratin, using fresh berries, follows. I like to serve this lukewarm, but it's good at room temperature as well—and it's good cold. Leftovers served right from the refrigerator make a splendid breakfast.

1 pound unsweetened frozen blackberries, thawed	3 tablespoons coarse dry whole wheat bread crumbs
2 heaping tablespoons brown sugar	1¼ cups low-fat fromage blanc or yogurt

1. Preheat the broiler to its highest setting.

2. Thoroughly mix the thawed berries with 1 tablespoon brown sugar and the crumbs. Spread the mixture into a nonreactive oval or round 2½-cup gratin dish.

3. Spread the fromage blanc or yogurt smoothly and evenly over the berries. Sprinkle the top with the remaining brown sugar.

4. Broil not too close to the heating element or flame for 4 to 5 minutes, until the mixture is bubbly and the sugar is caramelized. Allow to cool slightly. Spoon into glass bowls and serve.

FRESH BERRY GRATIN

Use whole raspberries, whole blueberries, halved strawberries, et cetera. The berries and part of the yogurt or fromage blanc remain cool, but the topping becomes hot and bubbly. It is a most pleasing contrast.

Berries	1 to 2 tablespoons dark brown sugar
Low-fat yogurt or fromage blanc	

1. Preheat broiler.
2. Spread the berries in a gratin dish.
3. Spread yogurt or fromage blanc evenly over the berries. Sprinkle evenly with the sugar.
4. Broil close to the heating element or flame for 1 minute, until the sugar is melted and bubbly. Serve *at once*.

RASPBERRY SAUCE

♡   *Makes 2 cups*

This is a basic dessert sauce, useful in myriad ways. It can top ice cream, or be swirled into fromage blanc or yogurt to create a fruit fool, or served as a dipping sauce for fresh whole strawberries.

Two 12-ounce packages frozen unsweetened raspberries, thawed and drained	**Sugar substitute to taste**

1. Purée the berries in a blender.
2. Pour the purée into a sieve and rub through. Discard the seeds.
3. Stir in the sweetener to taste. Refrigerate until needed.

🕐   Thaw berries in the microwave.

Variations:

Substitute other fruit—frozen black currants, strawberries, or blackberries—for the raspberries. Sweeten to taste. The Black Currant Sauce is wonderful enough to serve as a pudding all by itself (or perhaps topped with a dollop of low-fat yogurt or fromage blanc).

♡ ◔ # MANGO SAUCE

Place cubed, fresh, ripe mango (see Mango Sorbet, page 224, for procedure) into the jar of the blender. Purée until perfectly smooth. To end a summer meal on a sublime note, pour a puddle of Mango Sauce on each dessert plate. Heap a generous serving of raspberries on each puddle. Top with a cloud of Slim "Whipped Cream" (page 227). When raspberries are out of season, substitute peeled, sliced kiwi.

♡ ◔ # STRAWBERRIES ON RED AND WHITE SAUCE

This very beautiful dessert would make a perfect ending to a special dinner party. The Calories are minimal, but if the strawberries are good, it can hardly be bettered.

Fresh ripe strawberries	Buttermilk
Raspberry Sauce (page 229)	Mint leaves for garnish

1. Hull the strawberries.

2. Use clear glass plates, if possible. Pour some raspberry sauce on one half of the plate. Pour some buttermilk on the other.

3. Place the strawberries in a row down the dividing line. Garnish with fresh mint leaves.

CRUNCHY BANANAS ON RED AND WHITE SAUCE

♡

Serves 4

Kids love this, and adults won't complain either. The buttermilk, combined with the sauce, tastes deceptively rich and creamy.

1 heaping tablespoon low-fat
    yogurt or fromage blanc
1½ tablespoons dry whole wheat
    bread crumbs
	2 bananas
	Buttermilk
	Strawberry Sauce (page 229)

1. Preheat the broiler to its highest setting. Line the broiler pan with foil, shiny side up. Place a rack on the pan.

2. Put the yogurt or fromage blanc on a plate. Place the crumbs on another plate.

3. Cut each banana in half lengthwise. Cut each half into 5 pieces.

4. Dip the top side of each banana piece in the yogurt or fromage blanc, then dredge it in the crumbs. Place the dipped pieces on the broiler rack, crumbed side up.

5. Broil on the lowest rack for 3 to 4 minutes, until crispy on top.

6. For each serving, pour some strawberry sauce on half the surface of a small plate. Pour some buttermilk on the other half. Place 5 banana pieces down the center. Serve at once.

GINGER-LIME MOUSSE

♡

Makes 3½ cups

This mousse is exquisitely subtle and fragrant. Serve it to your gastronome friends as a finale to a very special dinner party. It's the sort of thing that should be eaten slowly and lingeringly, so that every nuance can be savored.

2 rounded tablespoons grated
   fresh ginger
Grated zest of 1 lime
Juice of 1 lime
1 envelope unflavored gelatin

¼ cup sugar substitute
2 cups low-fat yogurt or fromage
   blanc
1 cup buttermilk

1. Combine ½ cup water, the ginger, and the lime zest in a sauce-pan. Simmer for 5 minutes. Stir in the lime juice. Remove from the heat and stir in the gelatin. Let cool to room temperature.

2. When cooled, strain the mixture, pressing down on the solids to extract their flavor. Stir the sweetener into the strained mixture until it is dissolved.

3. Place the yogurt or the fromage blanc and the sweetened mix-ture into the container of the food processor, or blender. Process until perfectly smooth. While the machine is running, pour in the butter-milk in a steady stream.

4. Pour and scrape the mixture into an attractive serving dish or into 6 individual glass goblets. Chill for several hours or overnight.

APRICOT JAM

Makes 3 cups

1 pound dried apricots

2 tablespoons brandy

1. Put the apricots in a heavy saucepan. Add water to generously cover, and bring to a simmer.

2. Cover over low heat, stirring frequently, until the apricots lose their shape and cook into a lumpy mass. This will take anywhere from 15 minutes to 1 hour, depending on the fruit.

3. Stir in the brandy and a few more ounces of water. Cook for a few minutes more, stirring, until the mixture is very thick. Be careful not to let it scorch. Let cool.

4. Taste, and if the mixture is too tart, stir in a bit of sugar substitute

or sugar. If it's too sweet, stir in a few drops of fresh lemon juice. Scrape the mixture into a crock or bowl, cover tightly, and refrigerate. It will keep for weeks.

APRICOT CREAM

Fold together equal parts Apricot Jam (preceding recipe) and low-fat fromage blanc or "smoothed-out" drained cottage cheese. If desired, sprinkle each portion with a few toasted pine nuts.

STRAWBERRY CREAM FOR BREAKFAST OR TEA

     Makes 1⅛ cups

This is a splendid substitute for butter, Devonshire cream, or whipped cream and strawberry jam. Spread it on scones, bread, or toast for an unbelievably delicious low-Caloric snack. It tastes indulgent and luxurious, but contains just a fraction of the Calories of real cream and jam.

Very ripe or overripe strawberries	**A few grains of sugar substitute if**
Low-fat quark or "smoothed-out"	**necessary**
drained cottage cheese	

Mash the strawberries with a fork until their juices run. With a wooden spoon, beat the strawberries and their juices into the cheese. Sweeten to taste, if necessary. Scrape into a bowl or crock, cover with plastic wrap, and refrigerate for a few hours for the flavors to blend. This will keep for several days and improve in flavor each day.

ALMOND CURD WITH BLACK CURRANT SAUCE

Makes 3 cups

I borrowed the almond curd from Chinese cuisine, and added a dollop of fragrant Black Currant Sauce. The combination is stunning and deeply soothing.

1 envelope unflavored gelatin	¼ teaspoon pure vanilla extract
1½ cups hot water	6 tablespoons sugar substitute
1½ cups skim milk	Black Currant Sauce (page 229)
½ teaspoon pure almond extract	

1. Mix the gelatin into the hot water and stir until thoroughly dissolved. Stir in the milk and almond and vanilla extracts. Let cool to room temperature.

2. When cooled, add the sweetener, stirring until it is dissolved.

3. Pour the mixture into 4 to 6 glass dessert goblets and chill for several hours or overnight, until set.

4. To serve, top each serving with a dollop of Black Currant Sauce.

JELLIED TROPICAL FRUIT

Makes about 4 cups

This refreshing fruit gelatin is evocative of sunshine in both taste and color. It is a very soft fruit gelatin, not at all rubbery, so serve it in bowls, rather than trying to mold it. Passion fruit is ripe when it is wrinkled and wizened-looking; mango is ripe when it is soft to the touch and fragrant. It is impossible to say how much sweetener will be needed; it depends on the fruit and juices, so taste as you go.

3 cups fresh orange juice	Sugar substitute to taste
¼ cup fresh lime juice	4 passion fruits
2 tablespoons unflavored gelatin	2 ripe mangoes

1. In a saucepan, combine ½ cup orange juice with the lime juice. Sprinkle the gelatin over the juices. Stir over low heat until warm and the gelatin has dissolved. Do not let it come to a simmer.

2. Pour the remaining orange juice into a bowl. Stir in the gelatin mixture. Taste and add 1 tablespoon or so of sweetener, if the juice is particularly acidic. If the orange juice is sweet, you may need no sweetener at all, or only a sprinkle. Chill the mixture for 1 hour or so, until thickened but not set.

3. Meanwhile, cut the passion fruit in half, and scoop the pulp, seeds, and all into a blender container. Cut the mangoes in half (over a bowl, to catch the juices) and scoop out the flesh (see page 000 for procedure). Add the mango flesh and juices to the blender. Purée briefly. Push the purée through a nonreactive sieve to eliminate the passion fruit seeds.

4. Thoroughly stir the puréed mixture into the thickened juice. Taste and add sweetener, if needed. Stir thoroughly to dissolve.

5. Return the mixture to the refrigerator for another hour or so, until set. Serve spooned into glass goblets.

Variation:

Omit the passion fruit and use only mangoes, if desired. Instead of puréeing them, process them until they are finely chopped. Stir the chopped mangoes into the thickened juice in step 4.

INDEX

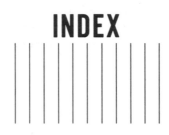

Carrot(s)
  baked, 29
  soup, 74–75
Casserole, frijol-albondiga, 101–103
Cast-iron frying pans, 45
Cauliflower
  braised, with fennel seeds, 173–74
  stir-"fried," 177
Cheese, 37–39
  "cream cheese," 21–22
  quark, 38–39
  on toast, 217
  See also names of cheeses
Cheesecloth, 46
"Chef's toque" symbol, 14
Chestnut soup, 82
Chicken
  bhuna, 142–43
  braised with garlic, 140–41
  breasts, 127
    curry, 136–37
    pan-sautéed, 128
    with raspberries, 134–35
    with yellow pepper sauce, 133–34
  chilaquiles, 145–46
  honey-mustard, braised, 139
  lasagna, 159–60
  legs and thighs, 128
  lemon-roasted, 146–47
  in onion-tomato gravy, 137–38
  oven-"fried," with mint dipping sauce,
    132–33
  poached, 144–45
  salad
    with berries, 129
    curried, 130–31
    molded, 129–30
  smoked, 35–36
    with penne and pesto, 164–65
  for stock, 31–32
  -tarragon pie, 143–44
  vindaloo, 141–42
Chicken stock
  basic, 31–33
  canned, 34–35
  chicken wing, 33–34
  Chinese restaurant, 34
  smoked chicken, 36
Chick-pea potato salad, 207
Chilaquiles, 145–46
Chili con carne, 113–14

Chili peppers, 41–42
Chinese bamboo steamers, 46
Chinese restaurant chicken stock, 34
Chinese style
  braised mushrooms, 184
  cabbage salad, 209
Clock symbol, 14
Club sandwich, 215
Cod en papillote, 95
Cooking techniques. See Techniques
Cookware, nonreactive, 45–46
Corn
  salad, 208–209
  soup
    chilled, 84
    Mexican, 84
Cottage cheese
  low-fat, 38
  "smoothed-out," 20–21
"Cream cheese," 21–22
Creams
  apricot, 233
  strawberry, 233
Cucumber
  raita, 203
  salad, marinated, 205
Curry(ied)
  chicken, 136–37
    salad, 130–31
  keema, 112–13
  kofta, 103–105
  roast potatoes, 196
  sautéed onions for, 18–19
  shepherd's pie, 110–11
  vegetable, 171–72

Dairy products, 36–39
Desserts, 221–35
  almond curd with black currant sauce, 234
  cream
    apricot, 233
    strawberry, 233
  crunchy bananas on red and white sauce, 230
  ginger-lime mousse, 231–32
  gratin
    blackberry, 228
    fresh berry, 228–29
  guidelines, 221–22
  ice cream, 222
    banana, 222–23
    banana-ginger, 223

| 240 |

10" enamaled cast iron fry pan